LOSE WEIGHT NOW!

*Vital Psychodynamics Programmes
to Lose Weight*

Antony Maurice-Nneke

Originally Published in 2011
NOW, fully revised including the additional entry of a formula to help with the success of Lose Weight Programmes and ways to deal with certain anxieties that might deter effort to lose weight.

First Published on Amazon Kendal 2023

British Library cataloguing in Publication Data

A catalogue record of this book is available from the British Library

ISBN: 9798393661908

By The Same Author

2023: Stop Smoking Now! Amazon Kendal

2022: Sex and Psychodynamics Psychiatry. Amazon Kendal

2013: Sex and Psychosexuality. Xianjian Press, China.

2003: The Psychodynamics of The Unconscious. Intapsy Pubs. London, UK

2002: Mind Castles. Intapsy Publications, London. United Kingdom

CONTENTS

ACKNOWLEDGEMENT

I thank my family for their support and for their general warmth and kindness towards me during my work on this book. I love you all.

INTRODUCTION

It is all in the state of mind, success in anything you do begins in the mind.

I.1 The Basic Idea of the Mind Technique in This Book

This book is a practical application of some of the ideas and fundamental principles of mind power technique that I introduced in my book, *Mind Castles* (2002).

The book presents a novel approach to weight loss and weight control which is simple, fun to practise and highly effective. It demonstrates a unique practical mind technique that enables the individual to lose weight steadily, easily, effectively and effortlessly. In doing so, the individual will look good and feel great.

The great advantage of this book is that it does not involve the reader in following any rigid fad diet. This book is not a dietary book or nutritional book. There are no diets to follow and the book is concerned mainly with losing the extra weight which was gained as a result of overeating as opposed to weight gain as a result of genetic problem, hormonal problem or the abuse of certain drugs such as steroids which can lead to massive gains in weight as used by body builders.

The book contains some of the essential secret weapons which an individual needs in order to look good and feel great in every way and realise, today, his or her body weight which he or she has always wished to be. The book teaches a special method of relaxation that enables the individual wishing to lose weight to make his or her dream weight a reality today.

When you practise the special method of deep relaxation that the book teaches, you may have the following feelings when you are relaxed..

- You may feel light and weightless.
- You may feel extremely relaxed in mind and body.
- You may feel as light and weightless as if you can just float away.

- You may have a feeling of joy and upliftment.
- You may feel a surge of power and energy with increased relaxation.

It is usual to have these feelings as by-products of your deep relaxation but they are not a necessary part of the application of this method of losing weight. What is necessary is that the individual must feel relaxed and be focused on the goal of losing weight.

However, if an individual can feel light and weightless during the moment of deep relaxation, he or she is beginning to lose weight mentally. This is the feeling which this book creates for individuals as they inculcate the habit of relaxation in the special way that is taught in this book. Refer to the prelude to the preparatory exercise in the next chapter to see one of the ways in which the feeling of weightlessness could come about.

When an individual has this feeling of weightlessness constantly in his or her mind, he or she will know that he or she is beginning to accomplish the goal of losing weight for success begins in the mind. The next stage is for the individual to translate the feeling into the physical activities that will make the feeling become his or her reality so that he or she can experience the weight coming off his or her body easily and effortlessly.

The simple mind techniques in this book are intended to enable any individual to harness the power to bring about the changes which he or she requires in life, be it in weight loss, giving up smoking, giving up alcohol, seeking for romance or in any other venture where the goal of the individual is to achieve success.

This book shows the way to achieve success in losing weight and it shows, truly, the way to achieve success in any goal or anything you do; how to be what you want to be, how to do things seriously in a positive way so that you do them successfully. It shows how to erect a solid foundation to the mind castles which many individuals build from day to day.

The strong message in the book is that you will get what you want when your mind is actively focused on what you want as a goal to be achieved. Any person who desires to lose weight would be successful in losing weight steadily, easily, effectively and effortlessly if the person has a positive mental attitude and a strong belief in his or her own ability to attain the desired weight steadily, easily, effectively and effortlessly.

The success comes through an intentional positive action as action is the route to change. Any person who can talk the talk about losing weight must walk the walk to realize the goal by putting the talk into action. This book is about responsible positive action which brings about positive changes by helping the individual to lose weight steadily, easily, effectively and effortlessly.

This book shows you how to inculcate a positive mental attitude, how to acquire self belief, self esteem and how to project a positive self image in whatever you do. The book takes you through the actions that you must perform, and the attitudes that you must adopt in order to achieve success in losing weight.

If you can bring yourself to believe that you have the power within you to lose weight, bring to reality a chosen weight that you can conceive as possible in your life, then you will be truly on your way to achieving your desired weight easily and effortlessly.

The conception of the possibility of the idea, and the reality of it, begin with effective thought bricks which form the foundation of your own mind castle in relation to losing weight steadily, easily, effectively and effortlessly. In this way, you will look good and feel great.

This idea will become much clearer to you in chapter one when I take you through the fundamental principles of the mind technique that I introduce in this book and combine this with your knowledge of the secrets of how the human mind works.

The claim of this book is that every individual has the power within him or her to accomplish whatever he or she wishes to accomplish in life, to make whatever changes he or she wishes to make in his or her life successfully. In order to do this seriously and conscientiously, the individual has to, first, acknowledge the enormous power within him or her and, secondly, make use of that power by doing something new or at least by doing something in a different way from before.

The emphasis here, as in 'walk the walk', mentioned above, is in positive action which consists in the diligent practise of the relaxation exercises in this book, doing something new or at least different from one's previous actions in order to accomplish one's goals and aspirations.

A person's acknowledgement and utilization of his inner power for success entails the belief that there is no limit to what he or she can accomplish, legitimately, with his or her mind except the limitations which he or she, wilfully, imposes on himself or herself by distorted thoughts and self doubt. The power of the mind is utilized in thought processes and this is manifested by an individual's actions in so far as thoughts precede actions.

By following all the positive ideas in this book and the actions that they invoke, the serious reader will develop a positive attitude towards the desired goal of losing weight. This will help him or her to lose weight steadily, easily, effectively and effortlessly. In this way, the reader will look good and feel great.

The reader will also develop a great confidence in his or her ability to succeed in any chosen venture and he or she will be ready, willing, and able to embark on the road to success. The essential ingredients that are required for a recipe for success in losing weight by the method of deep relaxation and vital mental programmes are in this book.

The effective use of these essential ingredients will propel any serious reader to the road of success in losing weight easily and effortlessly when he or she has read the book attentively from the beginning to the end and practised the techniques and the exercises diligently as advised in this book.

A person's decision to read this book brings that person a step nearer to the road of success in any venture. The person will be walking firmly on that road with the head held high by the time he or she has read to the end of this book. This will happen when he or she has read the book with concentrated attention.

Such attention must be supported by a clear understanding and performance of the necessary actions which an individual must take to achieve the success that he or she desires. Some of these actions consist in practising all the relaxation exercises for losing weight which are given in this book.

There is a clear user-friendly advantage to this book which is in the way that things look familiar to the reader as he or she reads through the pages of the book. This is partly because of the simplicity of the ideas, the relaxation exercises, and the way in which the ideas have been presented in this book and partly because the subject matter, *Losing Weight,* is a subject which is of great public interest. Many people seem to know someone else who they think needs to lose some weight.

In my work as psychodynamics analyst and lecturer in London, I organize regular seminars and workshops on mind power techniques such as techniques for memory to enable rememberance. This is particularly useful for examination candidates and test candidates of any nature. Also, techniques to stop smoking, and others. I have also worked in the area of sports translating the principles of depth psychology into the practical areas of sports performance.

I have used some of the simple mind power techniques discussed in this book to help my clients, many sports people such as athletes, boxers, footballers, gymnasts, and tennis players, to lose weight, stop smoking and to gain a great self confidence in what they do. This has enabled them to achieve success in their own sports by attaining a much desired personal best (PB) performance in their sports. These workshops are held regularly at various venues in London.

As a result of all these, I have every confidence in anyone reading this book for the serious purpose of losing weight. If this is your intention for reading this book, you must spend time to try out all the positive suggestions given and participate fully in the deep relaxation exercises given in *the practice sessions* in the book.

I.2 The Practice Sessions

This is a practical book for losing weight. As I mentioned above, if a person is able to talk the talk about losing weight, then that person must be prepared to put the talk into practical action and walk the walk which will lead him or her to the fulfilment of the desired goal. The *practice sessions* are an essential part of the positive action in this book and they are intended to help the reader to develop a relaxed attitude in mind and body. This will help him or her to focus the mind sharply on the desired objective of losing weight.

I.3 The Key Points to Remember

The key points to remember are given in the various sections of this book. They are quick reference to the issues raised in a particular discussion and provide a brief summary of the key points in the discussion. The act of remembering these key points forms part of the practical action in this book for one has to remember the ideas in order to put them into practice.

This book is in itself an exploration into the powers of the human mind. My underlying thesis is that success in anything we do begins in the mind. *It is all in the mind.* This becomes obvious as one reads through the pages of this book.

As I mentioned above, if you are reading this book with a serious intention to lose weight, you must practise the simple techniques in the book because simple techniques work. They work because they are simple. The simple techniques in this book are part of the simple techniques that I use every week in my own work and in the workshops that I organize.

I.4 Further Useful Secret Programmes in the Book

In addition to helping readers to learn how to lose weight steadily, easily, effectively and effortlessly, the readers will also learn the following secrets from reading the book.

- ❖ The secrets of how the human mind works.
- ❖ How to use effective thought bricks to erect an impregnable mind castle.
- ❖ How to relax and take control of any situation.
- ❖ How to recognise the effects of stress and anxiety in personal life.
- ❖ How to acquire confidence, self esteem and self worth.
- ❖ How to formulate goals and make plans for the future.
- ❖ How to make a plan of action to achieve a specific goal.
- ❖ How to visualise for success in any venture.

I.5 The Idea of Psycho-cybernetics

With reference to the above topics, you can also view this book as an introduction to psycho-cybernetics, the application of solid thought bricks as a foundation for the construction of mind castles in making radical changes in life.

In this respect, the book is a journey into a new world of positive possibilities, a new way of doing things, a new method of approach to personal and social problems, an adventure for self development and self improvement. I shall take you to a new experience in the world of positive possibilities in the next chapter.

I shall take you on a journey in the next chapter with a preparatory exercise to set the psychical system in motion so that you will feel relaxed. The preparatory exercise has a prelude to it which fixes it for you to be deeply relaxed and feel weightless. When you perform the prelude exercise and the main preparatory exercise properly, diligently, you will notice that you will feel relaxed in mind and body from that moment onwards.

CHAPTER ONE: ESSENTIAL PRELIMINARY STEPS TO LOSING WEIGHT

When you visualize something, you can make it a material reality. If you are able to visualize yourself in your chosen weight, the weight that you wish to be, and think constantly that you can lose weight and become your chosen weight, the weight that you wish to be, then this will certainly become your reality. This is the essence of visualization: whatever you visualize, you can realize it.

This book sets out to show you how to bring about the reality by the effective use of the powers of your mind. It takes you on a journey into a new world of infinite positive possibilities where all positive goals are fulfilled. Your goal to lose weight will be granted because it is a positive goal.

1.1 The Preparatory Exercises

Now come along with me to learn what to do as we begin the journey or quest for success in losing weight with a preparatory exercise. The preparatory exercise has two purposes to it. The first purpose is to prepare an individual for the regime of positive thinking and deep relaxation in mind and body by breathing through the diaphragm. The second purpose is to underline the role of visualisation in mental activities. A regular practise of the preparatoty exercise will enable you to feel relaxed constantly.

It is important to feel relaxed and be relaxed because with deep relaxation an individual can do things easily and effectively. With deep relaxation, your goal of losing weight will be accomplished easily, steadily, effectively and effortlessly. The preparatory exercise has two parts to it. The first part is a very potent but simple prelude to the main exercise, and the second part is the main exercise. I introduce them here as follows.

Prelude Exercise

As I begin to read this book and focus my mind on deep relaxation, peace and contentment, I feel deeply relaxed and as I count the numbers, slowly, now from ten down to zero, I will feel very light and weightless at the count of zero. I will feel as light and weightless as if I can float away. The count now is number ten, nine, eight, seven, six, five, four, three, two, one, going deeper and deeper and deeper all the way to z e r o. Now, I feel light and weightless, as light and weightless as if I can just float away.

As I continue to feel light and weightless in this way, I know that through the days and through the nights from this moment onwards the weights will drop off my mind and body steadily, easily and effortlessly and I will look good and feel great. In this way I will lose weight effectively and feel happy and contented that I have accomplished my goal easily and I have done so effortlessly.

Since I am thinking constantly about losing weight, the thoughts that I have constantly in my mind will materialize into reality for me, always. Thus, I will lose weight easily and effortlessly, look good and feel great.

Main Exercise

By practising the above prelude exercise or the main exercise below, the individual will inculcate the habit of relaxation so that it will become an everyday reality. In the main exercise below I shall take you on a journey to a world of infinite positive possibilities where all wishes are granted, all goals and desires accomplished and all dreams fulfilled. We shall proceed now on the journey through deep relaxation as follows.

Sit down comfortably on a chair or couch and let us start on our journey. Breathe in through your diaphragm. Hold your breath for a mental count of the numbers from five all the way down to zero. The count now is the number five, four, three, two, one, you are now going deeper and deeper all the way down to zero. Now, gently breathe out slowly and go deeper, deeper, deeper and deeper into relaxation.

As you are now relaxed, I want you to empty your mind of all doubts, all negative thoughts and mental distortions. Now, I want you to go deeper and deeper into relaxation as you imagine that you are listening to the sound of my voice so that with each word that I say to you, with each breath that you take and at each moment you are getting more and more involved with this exercise as your feeling of relaxation increases within your mind and body.

*I want you to learn that from this moment onwards the word **R E L A X** will bring instant relaxation to your mind and body so that whatever situation you are in, wherever you are, you will be absolutely relaxed and in total control, come what may.*

*Now, I want you to imagine that I am counting the numbers down to you, slowly, from ten all the way down to zero. As I count the numbers, you will go ten times more deeply relaxed and you will be relaxed on each and every descending number. Every number down will be a step to peace, tranquillity and total relaxation for you. The count now is the number ten, nine, eight, seven, six, five, four, three, two, one. You are now drifting, shifting down, down all the way to **z e r o.** You are now very, very, very deeply relaxed.*

I want you to know that some people have a tingling sensation when they are relaxed by this method, others have a feeling of elation, some others feel very light and weightless, as light and weightless as if they can float away, just as you felt in our prelude exercise a moment ago. A few other people feel heavy as they are laden with negative thoughts. At this particular moment whatever positive feeling you have is right and proper for you. So stay with your positive feeling as you go deeper, deeper and deeper into relaxation.

Now I want you to come with me for a journey to a new world. This is the world of infinite positive possibilities. It is a world of goodness, a world where you can do good deeds and achieve beneficial results and obtain whatever you want without harming or undermining other people.

In this world you can get whatever positive thing you want because whatever positive thing you want is what is available for you in the world of infinite positive possibilities. Every positive wish is granted and every goal is accomplished in this world. Your goal to lose weight is a positive goal which will be accomplished in the world of infinite positive possibilities.

There is an abundance of good wishes and beneficial things for everyone in this world. In this world all your wishes and desires are fulfilled. Your goals are accomplished in this world. You can lose weight easily, effectively, and effortlessly in this world of infinite positive possibilities because in this world everyone is a winner. Your journey to the world of infinite positive possibilities makes you a definite winner with your goal to Lose Weight Now!

Now before you make the journey I want you to spend a little time to deliberate on some of the serious health problems which are the effects of being overweight. As you are a health conscious person, you will notice that these health problems are the sound reasons which make it necessary for you to go on the journey to the world of infinite positive possibilities. The serious health problems are as follows.

- ❖ *Being overweight carries a risk of developing psychological depression.*
- ❖ *There are emotional and social problems attached to being overweight.*
- ❖ *There is a risk of heart problems in being overweight.*
- ❖ *Being overweight may lead to the threat of hypertension or high blood pressure.*
- ❖ *Overweight people may suffer from respiratory problems.*
- ❖ *Overweight people face the risk of developing gall bladder disease.*
- ❖ *Overweight people may suffer from arthritis.*
- ❖ *Overweight people may have problems with their immune system.*
- ❖ *Overweight people face the risk of developing Type 2 diabetes.*

❖ *Overweight people may be prone to stress and anxiety problems. They tend to appease these problems through food which, in turn, increases their weight.*

❖ *Overweight people may suffer from sweating problems.*

As you have taken the time to deliberate on the health reasons for losing weight, you are now very strongly aware of the health reasons for losing weight and the necessity for you to lose weight. As a result of these reasons, it becomes necessary that you must go to the world of infinite positive possibilities to lose weight steadily, easily, effectively and effortlessly. In this way you will look good and feel great, always.

You are now deeply relaxed, feeling peaceful, contented and ready to make the journey. Now, I want you to visualize yourself in a new world of infinite positive possibilities. I want you to be there at the count of the numbers from three down to zero. The count now is number three, two, one, drifting all the way to zero.

You are now in the new world of infinite positive possibilities. You can climb the highest mountain, parachute jump, bungee jump from the greatest height or accomplish a seemingly impossible feat in the world of infinite positive possibilities. Everything that is positive is possible in this world.

Every good wish and positive goal that you want to achieve is easily achievable in this world. Whatever positive goal or positive wish that you accomplish in the world of infinite positive possibilities will also be accomplished and retained by you in the actual world.

Everyone who gets to the world of infinite positive possibility becomes a winner instantly because everyone accomplishes a cherished goal in the new world of infinite positive possibility. You are already a winner for coming this far but you will stay with me to complete your time in this new world of infinite positive possibilities. You will stay in the new world of infinite positive possibilities for the time that it will take to accomplish your goal of losing weight and you will become a great winner.

Now, I want you to visualize yourself in the weight that you wish to be, the weight that you have chosen for yourself, and see yourself in what you regard as your correct weight and your correct size. I want you to stay with the knowledge that in the world of infinite positive possibility, you will accomplish your wish easily, and effortlessly.

Your positive belief, your optimism and the positive energy which you invest on your positive thoughts of losing weight will help you to accomplish your goal and any other wishes you might have. Now I want you to accomplish your goal of losing weight in the time that you have in the new world of infinite positive possibilities.

***This is your moment,** the moment of positive action and positive accomplishment, the moment of healthy attitude to eating and healthy living for you. You know what you have to do in order to let go the burden of carrying extra weight. You will act positively and lose weight accordingly. Do it now in this opportune moment.*

As you are now accomplishing your goal of losing weight, I will leave you for a moment for you to complete what you are doing and lose weight steadily, easily, effectively, and effortlessly. You will be successful in what you are doing and you will accomplish every positive desire that you wish to accomplish because every positive desire is granted in the world of infinite positive possibilities.

I will leave you now for you to accomplish your goal and when I return you will be deeply relaxed, well in control and happy with the knowledge that from this moment onwards you will be losing weight, steadily, easily, and effectively. You will lose weight effortlessly. Go on, do what you have to do in order to lose weight in the world of infinite positive possibilities and I will join you in a moment.

(I will Pause here briefly, for you to perform the exercise. Go on, you can do it)

You are now deeply relaxed. You feel peaceful and in control. You have done what you have to do and you have accomplished your goal of losing weight. You have done so, easily and effortlessly. Every other positive desire that you have is easily achievable by you from now onwards. Believe it for it is true.

Now as I count the numbers upwards from one to five, you will return to the world of actuality where you will actualize your goal of losing weight and every other positive desire that you have so that they become real accomplishments for you. At the count of five, you will be very deeply relaxed, confident, positive, very optimistic and in control. These feelings and attitudes will stay with you and be part of your everyday feelings and attitudes from this moment onwards.

The count now is number one, two, three, four, five. The number five has been counted. You are now in the world of actuality where you will actualize all your achievements from the world of infinite positive possibilities. If you had closed your eyes at the beginning of this exercise, you can open your eyes now and welcome to the actual world where you can realize your goals, wishes and desires.

NOTE

When you are giving instructions to yourself in relation to deep relaxation, you may count the numbers down to go deeper into relaxation. The higher the number from which you begin your count, the deeper you will relax as follows.

At the count of ten down to zero, you will be very deeply relaxed and in control. The count now is ten, nine, eight, seven, six, five, four, three, two, one, drifting, shifting all the way down to z e r o. You are now very deeply relaxed and in control.

Count the numbers upwards to come up, sit up and to open your eyes if they were shut for the exercise. In general, you may count up or down to perform a specific action in accordance with a specific instruction as follows.

At the count of one to five, you will open your eyes and sit up at the count of five with the knowledge that you are feeling light as the weights drop off your body steadily and effortlessly. The count now is one, two, three, four, five. You can open your eyes now and sit up.

When it is necessary to be deeply relaxed in order to perform a particular task, you may count the numbers down as follows.

At the count of ten down to zero, you will bring the warm, healing light of the sun over to your body and you will move it up and down your body to energise you and invigorate you at the count of zero. The count now is ten, nine, eight, seven, six, five, four, three, two, one, drifting and shifting all the way down to z e r o. Now bring the warm, healing light of the sun over to your body and feel it now as the healing rays of the light of the sun energises and invigorates you.

For the full force of this particular exercise, refer to chapter three where I make use of the light of the sun as a potent symbolism to bring peace, tranquillity, and positive accomplishments.

1.2 You Must Choose Your Weight

The objective of this book is to help you to lose weight. You will lose weight steadily, easily, effectively and if you focus your attention on deep relaxation as advised here, you will lose weight effortlessly because of the power of your unconscious mind which you will learn about here in this chapter.

In order that you lose weight steadily, easily, and effectively with the mind technique that I demonstrate here, it is advisable that you choose your own correct weight carefully. This is the weight that you wish to be, the weight that will make you feel comfortable. This will be the weight in which you will feel much more confident with yourself and your appearance. It is the weight in which you will look good and feel great about yourself generally.

You must exercise great care and caution in choosing your weight. Do not be hard on yourself by doing anything harsh or go to the extreme in your eagerness to lose weight. Some people lose weight so drastically that they become bean pole caricatures of their former selves. Remember, always, that there is as much health risk in acquiring the gaunt skeletal look as there is in being overweight.

I do not talk about 'ideal' weight and the mumbo jumbo of body mass index in this book as the burden of achieving an 'ideal' weight creates anxiety for some people as they get fixated on the problem of achieving an 'ideal' weight and fail to lose weight. This is because for some people an 'ideal' situation is usually a speculative, and unattainable situation.

The main objective in this book is to lose weight. This is easily attainable. It is to achieve success with the goal of losing weight and lose weight steadily, easily, and effectively, and to do so effortlessly by enlisting the aid of the power of the unconscious mind through the use of mental prompts.

The method of presentation in this book reminds you, constantly, of the fundamental principles of the mind technique, the secrets of the basic workings of the human mind, the power of the unconscious mind and the need for positive affirmation. This method is itself a potent mental prompt which sticks in your mind and helps you to keep your goal of losing weight alive. This makes your goal easily amenable to fulfilment.

Now, I want you to return to the exercises and the illustrations which I have given above. If you have performed the preparatory exercises and the exercises in the illustrations above about counting up and down, diligently and successfully, the other exercises in this book will become great fun for you because the above exercises set the pattern of the fun activities in this book.

The purpose of the journey to the world of infinite positive possibilities is to underline the role of visualization in mental activities. If you can visualize it, you can realize it, that is, make it real.

Visualization is a process by which an individual uses positive rational thought to create mental pictures of his or her goals, wishes or desires. The mental pictures help him or her to turn the goals, wishes or desires into reality. In short, visualization is the act of the construction of mind castles.

If you can bring thought and picture together about you losing weight and you are able to see yourself in the picture as you would like to be, you are conceiving a potent idea, building up something tangible, constructing mind castles. Any wishes, desires, intentions or major goals which you are able to conceive in this way, is easily achievable by you.

What you need to do next is to frame your mental picture to make it concrete. You require patience and the right mental attitude which will always be a positive mental attitude. This will help you to put a rock solid foundation to the castles which you have built in your mind.

However, you can also accomplish your goals, wishes, and desire even if you lack the ability to form mental images of what you want. It is sufficient to have an idea of what you want to accomplish and then bring it about through other means which are discussed here. A sound knowledge of the fundamental principles of the mind technique discussed here will help you immensely to accomplish any goal or desire. I said that you must **choose your weight.** This is an important part of your taking control of your lose weight programme.

1.3 The Fundamental Principles of the Mind Technique

Now I want you to come with me to begin the quest for success in losing weight right away by examining the fundamental principles of the mind techniques that I introduce in this book. The mind technique is a combination of the fundamental principles of the power of the mind and the secrets of how the mind works. These principles are the rock solid foundation to your mind castles and an understanding of them and an adherence to them will help you to understand what is involved in the use of the power of the mind to make positive changes in your life.

A constant adherence to these principles will enable you to accomplish your goals, wishes and desires. If you understand these principles and act on them constantly, then you will find that losing weight will be fun and easy for you.

In general, you will get what you want when your mind is deeply focused on what you want as a goal to be achieved. The mind techniques which are presented throughout this book are based on the general operation of the human mind in response to a certain belief of the individual.

Thus, in order to understand and master the practical mind techniques for losing weight easily, and effectively, it is essential that you understand the cardinal principles in the mind technique which I introduce here. Also, you will need to have a sound knowledge of the secrets of how the human mind works and the power of the unconscious mind. In what follows, I will show you the cardinal principles, the secrets of how the mind works, and the power of the unconscious mind.

If you are serious and sincere about your goals, you must apply this knowledge generally in your actions in order to achieve you goals and desires effectively. When this knowledge is applied constantly, the fundamental principles which are discussed here and the secrets of how the mind works will become part of the routine of everyday motor behaviour for the individual.

1. The Thought Bricks of the Mind

The thought bricks of the mind can either enhance an individual's power to lose weight or restrict the individual's effort to lose weight. Thoughts are the bricks with which we build our impregnable mind castles. In order to build castles in the air or on land, one needs solid and effective thought bricks to lay the foundation of the castle.

This principle of mind power stipulates that the most powerful or forceful thought of the individual is transformed into reality for the individual. This means that whatever thoughts you repeat powerfully and often enough will become realities for you.

The thoughts, whatever they are, which you have in your mind the most often will materialise into reality for you. For example, if you affirm or repeat constantly your thoughts of success in losing weight, you will achieve success in losing weight steadily, easily, effectively, and effortlessly. If you are thinking positive thoughts about your success in losing weight this will become your reality.

On the other hand, if you are preoccupied with self doubts and negative thoughts about what you want to do, constantly thinking about failures and difficulties, failure and difficulties will become your reality.

The general rule for the application of this principle is to have a positive mental attitude and think positive thoughts so that positive feelings will flow to you, automatically, which will lead you to the achievement of positive results in your life. Thoughts are the bricks of all building structures. Thoughts are in the mind. If your thoughts are all about success you will be successful, if you think mostly about failure, this will become your reality!

If you are always doubting yourself and doubting everything, you must remember that 'doubt' is a thought brick. If 'doubt' is the thought that you have most often in your mind, your 'doubt' will become your reality. Your doubt erases your positive thought and gives you the realisation of failure.

If you doubt your ability to lose weight and your doubt is the thought that you have most often in your mind, you will prove yourself right as a cowardly person who lacks the ability to believe in himself or herself. This will be shown clearly by your abject failure to lose weight inspite of careful guidance given here.

You will get what you think about for what you think about is what you get because thinking about it focuses your mind constantly on it and makes it easy for you to accomplish your objectives. Notice, in this respect, that the prelude exercise which you performed at the beginning of this chapter has this idea embedded into it.

You will lose weight easily and effectively if you think that you will lose weight easily and effectively and believe from now onwards that you will lose weight easily and effectively because this is why you are reading this book. Your belief in the idea of success is a positive thought that stirs your mind to positive efforts and leads you to success. Negative thoughts and self doubts dampen the edge of positive action because they stir your mind away from your chosen objective and thus, lead you to failure and disappointment.

This first fundamental principle of the operation of the mind is vital in everything that we do, the plans and the decisions that we make from day to day. The operation of this first principle is embodied in the functions of the unconscious mind which I will discuss below in this chapter. If what you want to do is not quite clear in your mind, one way to tackle it is to see the problem as a challenge which must be confronted. In this way you will be inspired to investigate the solution and find out more about it.

If your reaction to a problem is negative and you adopt a negative attitude just for the purpose of avoiding the problem or, if you run away completely from the problem, you may find that you will be running away each time you perceive something as a problem; you will not solve any problem by running away from it. Thus, if the supposed problem concerns your goals and aspirations, then it is clear that the goals will not be achieved by running away from them.

Please do not misunderstand the points about your thought bricks. It is natural to have doubts about things that are unclear. The central point here is that you should not allow your doubt to be the only thought brick that you have on your mind. If you must have a doubt in relation to your goal, let your doubt be a methodical doubt which will lead you to investigate the source of doubt.

Please do not allow your doubt to lead you to run away from a perceived problem or give up on a goal which you have chosen. Always remember that giving up on a goal because of doubt or fear would only guarantee failure and disappointment to you in terms of the goal.

2. There is a Limitless Intrinsic latent Power within Everyone
The power of the human mind is awesome. It can bring great results when it is used in a positive way and it can cause enormous amount of problems, disaster and ruin when used in a negative way. I want you to understand that the power of your mind is potentially unlimited, that is, you have an unlimited potential within you now to accomplish anything you wish and to achieve positive results in your life, including the power to lose weight steadily, easily, effectively, and effortlessly. In this way you will look good and feel great.

There is no limit to the power of your mind except those limitations which you wilfully impose on your mind by yourself through negative thoughts. The power of the human mind is ingenious and prodigious. The ingenuity of the human mind enables humans to design sophisticated computers but, the power of your mind is much greater than that of the most sophisticated computer because the computer is designed by human mind and it is, by itself, unoriginal.

The power of your mind is there with you throughout your life from the moment of your birth. You can control your entire life with your mind. The magic of success in anything you do is within you. It is within your mind. Your mind is the magic power through which you achieve great success in whatever you do.

The essence of this second principle is that acknowledging the prodigious power of your mind will help you to lose weight easily and effectively because, with increased deep relaxation, the simple mental programmes in this book are easily assimilated in your mind as you read this book. Your mind has the natural ability to record all the mental prompts given throughout this book from the preparatory exercises to all the other exercises in the book and it will make this a part of your everyday motor action.

3. The Principle of Universal Energy
There is a universal energy within everyone. You can channel this energy to your desired goals and aspirations by way of your belief and attitudes toward your goals. As in the points which I made above, positive attitudes toward your goals channel positive energy to you. This leads to the successful fulfilment of your goals and aspirations. In the opposite way, negative attitudes and self doubts channel negative energy to you. This leads to failure, lack of fulfilment, and disappointment.

The energy which you put forth and the energy which you attract combine to determine the success or failure of your goals. Your attitude towards your major goals, your immediate objectives, and your life in general have a great impact on what you desire to create for yourself and to the extent, degree or urgency of your desire, on account of the energy invested on them.

The essential question for you here is how to determine what may need to change or evolve within you in order to transform you into a powerfully attractive force of energy. This will help to bring about the things that you focus your mind deeply on, desires and goals such as lose weight now into reality.

You can manifest your goals and desires more effectively by channelling positive attitudes towards them with greater expectation of their realization. In other words, the energy of your belief helps to make reality of your goals. Refer also to the first principle above.

In our everyday motor activities, each one of us channels his energy as dictated by his attitudes, feelings and beliefs in order to obtain the results he or she requires. Although occasionally, unfortunately, it happens that the energy of the individual is channelled negatively and the individual obtains the result that he or she does not require. You know already how this is likely to happen from our discussion above about the power of the first principle of our mind technique, the thought bricks of the mind.

The universal energy which is in everyone can also be manifested in a different way in every action of the individual because the individual attracts energy and also radiates energy into the universe by his attitudes towards events and situations in his life. Positive attributes such the possession of abundant wealth and prosperity, happiness, a person's success in achieving a particular goal, romantic bliss, developing rock solid absolute confidence in one's self, possessing positive feelings are all manifestations of this energy.

On the other hand, negative attributes such as failure in any venture, lack of confidence, negative feelings and other bad feelings are also manifestations of this energy.

Other ways in which the energy can be manifested, for example, feeling undermined, rejected, and alone, feeling inferior, feeling unworthy for success and so forth. All the ways to manifest the energy are within you because the energy is in you. The energy can manifest success, happiness, prosperity and abundance much easier than it can manifest failure and destitution because the natural state of the universe is for happiness, prosperity and abundance.

There is also a central dynamic pure energy force of magnetic power of creativity which is within everyone. The knowledge of this inner magnetic power within you should enable you to change the pattern of your thought and belief system and make them beneficial for you. You can do great things and achieve great goals if you believe that you have a dynamic, pure energy force of magnetic power within you to attract the things you wish in life by your attitudes and your actions.

The potent thought brick here within this principle is that you are a magic magnet, a centre of the magnetic power in the universe and that everything that you desire, your goals and aspirations are irresistibly drawn to you. This indwelling power in you guarantees that you can lose weight because you believe that you can. You can turn your belief into an affirmation and affirm your success in losing weight as follows.

I am a magic magnet. I am the centre of the magnetic power in the universe. My success in losing weight is irresistible drawn to me. I will lose weight easily and effortlessly because the magic of success is truly within me and it is evident in my magical magnetic powers.

This idea that what you desire, your goals and aspirations are irresistibly drawn to you by the magnetic force of your belief is an essential doctrine in depth psychology and it entails the belief that if you think that you can do it, you can. If you believe that you can lose weight, so be it, you can. The force and energy of your belief engenders positive action to realize your wish. This book teaches you to believe that you can, and to always believe that you can.

You can see quite clearly from what I have been saying here about energy, that success in anything, success in losing weight steadily, easily, effectively, and effortlessly is within your grasp because the energy to generate success is in you. Success in losing weight steadily, easily, effectively, and effortlessly is a universal energy which is an integral part of your natural power.

Success and wealth are external expression of abundance but the energy of abundance which causes the success and wealth to manifest in your life is internal. Thus, you can see from this that the magic of success is truly in you. Your success in losing weight now is within you.

4. Every Individual is the Architect of his own Life

Every, adult, individual is responsible for the state of affairs of his or her own life. As a result of an individual's thought patterns in general he or she is responsible for the way and manner he or she makes progress or failure on this planet in respect of the choices and decisions that he or she makes according to how and where his or her thoughts lead to in the execution of a particular action.

It is not right for a man to defend himself for his failures and lack of progress at any venture by finger pointing, blaming the state, other people, or by blaming God in appealing to the arguments of determinism, predestination, or fatalism. It is, equally, not right for a woman to do so.

You have the freedom to change your life by changing the pattern of your thoughts in making them more positive and beneficial to you. This is an essential principle of the power of the mind. You are the architect of your life and you can change your life by changing the pattern of your thoughts.

To profit from this principle, you have to proceed by seeking for ways in which you can take complete control of your life. Develop your creative ideas by making them more beneficial to you. Avoid the temptation to finger point and blame other people. Endeavour to become more and more assertive and self-reliant, and less and less dependent on other people for assistance.

Take full responsibility and draw out a plan of action for losing weight and follow the ideas given in this book, perform all the exercises in this book and settle on the one that makes you feel more comfortable.

5. Action is the route to change.
Your action is an expression of your thought. This is why a devious action is often condemned as a thoughtless action. The principle of positive action which I mentioned above is an essential ingredient in a recipe for success in any goal. If it matters to you then the onus is on you to do something about it. If you are truly convinced that you need to lose weight then you must take action to do so and lose weight now! In doing so, you will look good and feel great.

In your actions, you must always act with conviction. If you are giving a positive message to yourself or reading out your own affirmations, you must always act with the conviction that your message is going to be received by your unconscious mind and that your wishes and intentions will be realised, that is, made real.

The essential maxim for action which you must always remember is in what I said above under the second principle that if you think you can, you can. If you believe that you can do it, you can. No one is ready for success in any venture unless he or she believes that he or she can achieve it.

This is an incontrovertible thesis of the power of the mind. Always endeavour to be enthusiastic in what you do and act with absolute faith in your expectation of success. This part about your expectation is also included in your manifestation of the energy to bring about the desired result. Refer to the affirmation which you made, above, about your magnetic power.

Always avoid the temptation to fall into the negative pattern of blaming other people, for example, your partner, the government, the food manufacturers or the supermarkets when things go wrong in your attempt to lose weight. Take responsibility for your own affairs and do something about it by taking positive action to effect desired changes in your life.

With respect to our first principle which is a cardinal thesis of the power of the mind, it is important to realise that the power of thought is the essence of the mind. The influential French philosopher Rene Descartes (1596-1650) saw this during his great meditations which led him to assert his famous maxim, *Cogito Ergo Sum* (I think, therefore, I am) in his writings, *Discourse on Method* (1637) and *Meditations on First Philosophy* (1641). Descartes saw the exercise of *thinking* as the indubitable proof of an individual's existence.

The operation of thinking is a function of the mind. The thinking power of the mind is clearly illustrated in all the deliberations and cogitations which Descartes went through in his meditations and all his other ruminative activities in order to establish the certainty of the *Cogito*. Descartes could have equally said, *Credo Ergo Sum* (I believe, therefore, I am) as a strong belief is important in arriving at the result that you require. Remember that belief is also a thought brick. Refer to the first principle above.

In order to acquire the technique of mind power and be able to build effective mind castles, you must always be able to apply the above fundamental principles of mind power generally in everything that you do in your everyday life with respect to your thinking patterns with regard to whatever projects or goals you have. For the particular purpose in this book, the project or goal is losing weight. The fundamental principles mentioned above are applied in the techniques which I discuss in this book together with the secrets of how the human mind works.

1.4 Key Points to Remember

- ❖ Your thoughts are the bricks for mental constructions. Positive thoughts give solid foundation to your building projects and help you to lose weight easily and effortlessly. Negative thoughts dampen the edge of positive action, lead to failure, destruction, disappointment, and ruin.
- ❖ The power of your mind is limitless. Acknowledging this power enables you to know that you can achieve whatever you put your mind to. Thus, the magic of success in losing weight is

truly within you, it is in your positive acknowledgement of the principles which I have discussed above in relation to your thoughts about losing weight.

❖ There is a universal energy within you which manifests success or failure according to your thought patterns in relation to your goal of losing weight.

❖ You are the architect of your own life. You have the power to effect changes in your life because it is up to you, not other people.

❖ Acknowledge that you have the power of a dynamic creative energy force within you which, when recognised, enables you to bring about positive changes in your life.

❖ The power of your mind is greater than that of the most sophisticated computer because the computer is created by the ingenuity of the human mind.

❖ Remember that action speaks louder than words and act positively to bring about the changes which you seek because action is the route to change.

1.5 The Secrets of How the Human Mind Works

I will now explain to about how the mind works by examining the levels of mental awareness, or the levels of consciousness, if you like. The advantage of this is that by knowing how the mind functions you will be in a better position to direct our thoughts to greater, more beneficial, purposes and achieve the results that you desire. This will help you to programme your actions more effectively with appropriate mental prompts to help you to lose weight steadily, easily, effectively and effortlessly. In this way, you will look good and feel great.

An individual's knowledge of how the mind works will enable the individual to appreciate the powers of his or her memory as a facet of the mind and then to achieve the result that he or she desires by using his or her memory to his or her own advantage. I am concerned here with the quality of consciousness in psychical topography.

When you read this book with a serious intention to lose weight you will find, very quickly, that the deep relaxation exercises and the positive mental prompts in the book will become part of your memory which is, in this respect, your unconscious mind. This is where the ideas need to be in order to form part of your motor activity.

The human mind functions at three principal levels. These levels have been clearly recognised within the field of depth psychology, that is, the psychology of the dynamic forces in the interaction between conscious and unconscious mental processes. These levels are more appropriately perceived as levels of mental awareness. They are as follows.

The Conscious Level
This is the level of everyday waking life. You are now reading this book at the conscious level of your mental functioning if you are aware that you are reading this book and know fully well that you are reading it and why you are reading it. At the conscious level the mind functions well when one is awake and so at this level one is able to reason, analyse, criticise, and control voluntary action. Your decision to lose weight and your decision to read this book and use it for losing weight are both made at this level, the conscious level of mental awareness.

The Preconscious Level
This is the level of latent ideas which are capable of becoming conscious at anytime. For instance, there were certain things which happened to you yesterday, last week, last month or last year and some other things which you caused to happen yesterday, last week, last month or last year in so far as their occurrence was the direct result of your own action.

As I have now got your undivided attention because you are listening to me, attentively, at this moment in reading this book, your mind is not concentrating on the events of yesterday, last week, last month or last year because it is occupied with the events of the moment in listening to what I am saying to you.

However, since I have now provoked you or stirred up your mind by mentioning the events of yesterday, last week, last month or last year, the flow of thoughts of those events may now come to your mind without difficulty because they have been triggered by my reference to them.

Those memories that have now been triggered by my reference to them are said to be at the preconscious level of mental functioning because they are latent memories which are at the threshold of consciousness. They are not being used at any moment, though they are not forgotten.

The Unconscious Level
This level was first investigated as a way to understand the power of the mind and the basis for the treatment of mental disorders by the Viennese neurologist and physiologist, Sigmund Freud (1856-1939), founder of psychoanalysis. The unconscious level is the most confused and confusing level of mental functioning. Freud described psychical topography in his article 'The Unconscious' (1915) in his collective works *On Metapsychology: The theories of Psychoanalysis*. For the purpose of the technique for losing weight which I introduce to you here, the theory of the unconscious consists of the following.

- ❖ The idea of the inaccessibility of mental items to consciousness due to their repression.
- ❖ The belief that such mental items which are inaccessible are, at the same time, causally active. Unconscious items have the power to affect the individual by giving rise to psychoneurotic symptoms and other puzzling or embarrassing behaviours whose origins have escaped the individual's consciousness because of their repression which makes them inaccessible.
- ❖ The belief that unconscious materials belong to a general psychical system of unconsciousness to which all unconscious materials inhere. This general psychical system is described by Freud as the *system unconscious*.
- ❖ Memories which are stored in the unconscious remain there permanently until released by the individual, either through the method of deep relaxation which I shall be teaching you here with illustrations or through abreaction during the process of therapeutic analysis.

However, for the purpose of your understanding of the power of the mind, your own unconscious mind is the simple and uncomplicated part of your mental awareness at which your mind is deeply relaxed and is totally uncluttered by bias, criticism, self doubt, tension, general disbelief or any disturbing emotions.

At the unconscious level the mind faithfully records, reproduces and controls the entire sensory and motor activities of the individual. By this I mean that the unconscious level controls all the general processes of thought bricks that provoke an individual's actions and other motor activities.

In this respect, every experience of an individual's life, every feeling, reaction, emotion and so on is recorded in the unconscious level of an individual's mind and can be reproduced during moments of deep relaxation. The unconscious is seen, in this sense, as the reservoir of everything that happens in an individual's life and everything that constitutes the individual's personality.

The unconscious is the totality of an individual's character and attitudes, the storehouse of all memory, and the centre of all the individual's habits. I have described this view of the unconscious elsewhere as the *container theory of the mind* (Maurice-Nneke 2003).

In his book, *The Structure and Dynamics of the Psyche, Collected Works, Volume 8,* the Swiss psychiatrist, Carl Gustav Jung (1875-1961), founder of the Society of Analytical Psychology and former sidekick of Sigmund Freud, describes the unconscious as a "receptacle of all memories".

With respect to losing weight the unconscious level of the mind functions in an automatic way, recording and reproducing the events of an individual's life. All beliefs, thoughts, feelings and so on are stored or recorded in the unconscious, the everlasting receptacle and these are reproduced automatically in the individual's thoughts and motor actions.

For example, here is my first illustration of the power of the unconscious and its effect on the lives of people. If a person has negative thoughts and believes that he or she might fail with his or her goal of losing weight such belief is stored or recorded in the person's unconscious and reproduced in his or her motor actions. Such a person will not take a positive action to lose weight because he or she believes that such action will be a failure.

Thus, failure will become his or her reality because he or she thinks about failure. In other words, a person who has a negative attitude towards his or her goal will find that the negative attitude will be recorded in his or her unconscious mind and failure will become his or her reality. In this illustration, you can see that 'failure' is the dominant, powerful, thought that the individual has most often in the mind. Thus failure becomes the individual's reality. Refer to the first fundamental principle which I discussed on section I.3 above.

On the other hand, if the individual has positive beliefs about himself or herself, his or her goals and aspirations about losing weight and attaining the correct weight which the person has chosen, the weight that the person wishes to be, these are what will be recorded in the unconscious and they will come true for him or her. This will help him or her in the achievement of positive results in life and accomplish a desired objective.

The unconscious level controls involuntary action and it is very receptive and active during sleep and in waking state. Remember the first principle of mind power, what you think of most often becomes your reality. This is because what you think of most often is what is recorded in the unconscious mind.

At the unconscious level all rational thought are suspended. Thus at this level, the mind does not reason, analyse, or criticize. Instead, all thinking processes which are carried out at the conscious level are stored up and played back in the unconscious. Thus, when ideas and beliefs are recorded in the unconscious, whether false or true beliefs, the mind retains them automatically and the ideas, beliefs, thoughts, or feelings are acted out by the individual in motor activity.

This is how your thoughts become your reality. This is how it is possible for you to lose weight easily and effectively. The positive ideas contained in this book will be acknowledged by your unconscious mind as you read these pages with positive feeling, confidence, and optimism about your success in losing weight. Your positive feeling, confidence, and optimism will enable the ideas to be retained by your unconscious mind to be acted out in your motor activity.

With respect to this power of the unconscious, you can see clearly from what I have said here that when positive ideas about success in losing weight are recorded in the unconscious, the individual automatically thinks positively about achieving success in losing weight and in whatever venture he or she engages in.

However, when negative ideas are recorded in the unconscious in relation to the ideas of the subject or venture, the individual shies away from the subject or venture and procrastinates and vacillates about the right things to do or the most appropriate goals to have and ends up with nothing because he or she is unable to decide.

As a matter of information, the term *unconscious*, as described above and used throughout this book, is the correct name for what you, probably, know as the 'subconscious'. The term 'subconscious' implies an inferior state and does not give an adequate description of the dynamics of mental processes. On the contrary, the unconscious is the most powerful force in the dynamics of mental functions. If you wish to know more about the unconscious, refer to my more elaborate book on the subject (Maurice-Nneke 2003).

The Supraconscious Level
There is a fourth level of mental awareness known as the *supraconscious* level. This is responsible for direct knowing and it functions independent of ordinary thought processes. It is utilised for extrasensory perception (ESP). ESP is a term which is used to describe four areas of mind power. These are the powers of clairvoyance, precognition, psychokinesis (also known as telekinesis), and telepathy.

Clairvoyance is the power to specifically perceive or know an event or object that is out of the natural range of human knowledge or perception, without the use of ordinarily recognised means of human knowledge or perception. *Precognition* is the power of the knowledge of future events in advance of their occurrence without deducing their occurrence from available data. *Psychokinesis* (PK) or *Telekinesis* (TK) is the power to use the mind to cause motion and changes in external objects. *Telepathy,* also known as thought transference, is the power of direct mental communication between two persons who may not necessarily be at close quarters.

A person who is adept in the use of any of these powers of the mind is usually described as *psychic* and the four areas of mind power constitute what is called *psi* (referring to psychic power). However, the term *psi* is also the name of the 23rd letter in the Greek alphabet. This term is usually employed in theories, equations, and experiments to denote an unknown quantity as opposed to what is given or postulated.

Thus, to the world of natural science psi, as denoted by the four areas of mind power given above, is still an unknown quantity despite decades of psychical research by eminent parapsychologists in Britain and the USA. This is not totally surprising because natural science is slow to open up to ideas outside its limited boundary and it is opposed to the existence of the mind. Many scientists, as scientists, disdain the idea of the psychical or the mental. They believe that everything is physical. As individuals, however, they may admit to themselves that mind exists otherwise they make no sense when they use the expression 'I have a mind of my own'.

Many people today still scoff at an individual's manifestation of any psi power as they did in the past. For example, during his time with Freud before his resignation from the International Psychoanalytic Association, Carl Gustav Jung dabbled in psychic activities and tried to impress Freud by showing his psychokinetic powers to Freud. However, Freud as a man of science, scoffed at it, described Jung as a mystic and questioned the scientific validity of mysticism and ESP powers. For more information about Jung and mysticism refer to my earlier book (Maurice-Nneke, 2003) and Jung's book, *Memories, Dreams, Reflections* (Carl Gustav Jung, 1995).

Even today in the new millennium ESP power is still looked at with disapproval in some quarters. Thus, those who possess some of the ESP powers described above only advertise their craft in the back pages of astrological publications and esoteric magazines.

Some people are very sceptical. They doubt that the clairvoyants possess any real powers of vision and still regard them as charlatans. Some other people wear the 'It's not scientific' (INS) cloak. This is an imaginary cloak of intellectual smugness which confers an illusory sense of superiority to those who wear it while, at the same time, it betrays their lack of knowledge and understanding of the particular subject of enquiry. Such people find it difficult to give credit to what they are unable to understand or explain scientifically. Thus, they embarrass themselves by seeking refuge in their own limitations of knowledge.

I am not saying that you should endorse the psychics if you have doubts about their claims. I believe that if you have genuine doubt, your doubt should provoke you to investigate the topic of doubt further, if only for the purpose of proving yourself right. I am saying, very strongly, that you should only doubt any claim if you have constructive arguments to refute the claim. Merely saying that something 'is not scientific' is not a refutational argument.

I firmly believe that a truly educated person is one who has an open mind to the things that he or she does not understand and cannot explain. Things do not become rubbish, silly, or stupid just because one lacks the experience or the intellectual ability to understand them! Always remember the dictates of the following maxim.

"There are more things in heaven and earth, Horatio,
Than are dreamt in your philosophy".
(William Shakespeare, *Hamlet* Act 1, Scene 5)

On the surface, ESP powers are not directly relevant to losing weight. However, a person who has ESP powers uses the energy forces as mentioned in the fundamental principles above and such a person could apply the ESP powers in the exercises for losing weight which are given in this book. The clairvoyant could foresee the success of the goal to lose weight and telekinetic exercises could be channelled to all the relaxation exercises given in this book and used to adjust the body to the chosen weight, the weight that the individual wishes to be.

1.6 Key Points to Remember

There are four levels of mental action

- ❖ The Conscious level is the level of everyday waking life, the level at which you are reading this book now.
- ❖ The Preconscious level is the level of latent memories which can be recalled at any moment without difficulty.
- ❖ The Unconscious level is the level of memories which have been repressed and have become inaccessible to the individual.
- ❖ The Supraconscious level is the level of great natural creativity, inspirational work and the power of the mind for extrasensory perception.

1.7 Belief as an essential ingredient in losing weight

Belief, like action, is an essential ingredient in a recipe for success in anything you do. It is an attitude of mind which encompasses everything you do in relation to the objectives you wish to accomplish.

There is an enormous power in believing. A man or woman can achieve a seemingly impossible goal, perform the greatest feat and achieve a personal best (PB) performance in competitive sports when he or she believes in the possibility of accomplishing the goal. A man's belief or conviction has an effect on the way he lives his life because it can make the difference between success and failure. You can lose weight now, easily and effortlessly if you strongly believe that you can. Remember the positive possibilities in your journey to the new world in our preparatory exercise at the beginning of this chapter and have the idea of the possibility of success in your mind always.

Belief can be positive or negative. Each form of belief affects the individual differently. A positive belief is a detergent to doubt. A positive belief that you will lose weight now stirs your mind to positive action and enables you to lose weight steadily, easily, effectively, and effortlessly. A belief that you would not be able to lose weight, that it is all a waste of time, is a negative belief. This form of belief blunts the edge of positive action and leaves you incapable of accomplishing your objectives. A negative belief in relation to your goal leads disastrously to failure.

A negative belief fans the flames of doubts and panders to idleness. Both positive and negative beliefs are ways of channelling your energy to your objectives or goals. The positive energies bring success to you while the negative energies bring failure and disappointment to you. In order to understand this properly, you must refer to the principles of mind power which I discussed above at the beginning of this chapter.

1.8 You Must Have Total Belief and Faith in Yourself

In another sense belief is an attitude of mind which encompasses everything you do in relation to what you wish to achieve. The power of belief is in its usage; it is not something which you possess and leave at home in your briefcase or something which you leave in a box, cupboard, or in your pocket. Belief is something about you which lies in the power within you in expressing your attitudes and opinions in everything you do to achieve your objectives. Belief, like confidence, is the way you carry yourself strongly, forcefully, in your actions, attitudes, opinions and behaviours from day to day.

There is a strong sense in what I have said above, in which belief refers to absolute trust or confidence. This is the sense in which I use the word **belief** in this book. It is the sense in which someone may say 'I believe in God' or the sense in which it may be said to someone that, 'You must have total belief in yourself'.

This sense of belief is like **faith**, an absolute, confident trust in the truth, value, efficacy, or worthiness of the ideas or plans which you hold on a given subject matter project of enquiry or venture. Belief is, in this sense, very essential for success because it enhances your powers of persistence. You must understand in this sense that no one is ready for success in any goal or venture until he or she believes that he or she can achieve success in the particular goal or venture.

You must have absolute faith and trust in yourself and in what you are doing in order to succeed in your venture. Belief is the opposite of doubt. When you have belief you are able to pursue your goals without doubting your ability to succeed in them. In order to understand this much better you must refer to my discussions above of the fundamental principles of the mind power technique in this book.

What is pertinent for the present purpose of losing weight is that those beliefs which a person, mistakenly, takes as knowledge are recorded permanently in the unconscious mind. These affect the person's attitude in relation to the things that matter in his or her life.

A false and negative belief in relation to losing weight and the achievement of success will cause a person to have twisted ideas about losing weight. These twisted ideas must be eradicated and replaced with positive ideas backed up with belief for the individual to achieve success with the goal of losing weight or with any other goals of the individual.

Belief is the essential ingredient in a recipe for success in whatever you do, you must have total belief in yourself and in whatever venture you wish to embark on in order to succeed in it. You must have an unwavering, rock solid, absolute belief in yourself and in your ability to lose weight steadily, easily, effectively, and effortlessly.

Some people start by doubting themselves. They want success but they think about failure so what they think about materialises for them. They ask, "What if it fails?" If they are concentrating on failure, it will be their reality. The appropriate questions will be about success.

Remember that if you are already thinking of failure before the start of your goal or venture, you will be working hard to give yourself the guarantee of failure and failure will become your reality.

Refer to the fundamental principles of the mind power technique and my discussions above about the secrets of how the human mind works and, in particular, try to understand the power of the unconscious mind as I have discussed above.

It is good to recognise your weaknesses on certain issues. This is positive thought brick and part of reality testing. It will lead to positive plans of action on how to improve those weaknesses. It will help the individual to make necessary improvements in the area of weaknesses so that one would be stronger, generally. However, recognising one's weaknesses is distinct from doubting one's ability to do something because while one leads, positively, to self improvement, the other leads, negatively, to the avoidance of the topic or subject of doubt and, thus, to failure and disappointment..

1.9 Key Points to Remember

- ❖ Belief is the essential ingredient in a recipe for success in any venture.
- ❖ You must have total belief, a rock solid, absolute faith in yourself in order to be successful in whatever you do.
- ❖ Belief is the opposite of doubt. When you have belief you pursue your goals without doubts about your chances of success.
- ❖ Remember that no one is ready for success in any goal or venture until he or she believes that he or she is capable of achieving success in the particular goal or venture.

1.10 How to Eliminate the Negative Power of Self Doubt

Remember that belief is the opposite of doubt. Do not defeat yourself by doubting yourself before you start. Do not place unwanted barriers on your path to success through relentless but unnecessary doubts. Self doubt shows insecurity, lack of esteem and lack of faith in your ability to achieve success with your goal. If you lack faith in yourself how would you expect others to have faith in you?

The way to get out of the negative, defeatist, thinking trap is to break down the negative thought patterns that restrict you from making essential progress in your chosen field. Whenever negative thoughts flow to your mind in relation to your ability to lose weight, you must start to cancel out the negatives by thinking positive thoughts about the possibility of attaining your desired weight steadily, easily and effectively. Remember your journey to the world of infinite positive possibilities. When you visualize your success you will be able to realize it, that is, make it real.

Whenever you feel positive about what you are doing or about what you are about to do, you will know that you will be successful in it. Whenever you think positive thoughts about your goals and aspirations, positive feelings will flow to you, automatically.

Each time you introspect about the good things that have happened to you in your life, you will feel positive right away. Whenever you think about all the goals that you have achieved in the past till now, you will feel positive immediately.

Whenever you think positive thoughts about your life in general, you will feel positive straightway. When you think about the positive effects of losing weight steadily, easily, effectively, and attaining the weight which you have chosen for yourself, the weight which you would like to be now, positive feelings flow to you automatically!

You will find that as you concentrate your thoughts in this way, positive feelings will flow, automatically, to you. *Think positive thoughts and positive feelings will flow to you, automatically.* It works every time. Try it **NOW** and see what happens. Go on and try it now even as you read this book. You will feel positive instantly. Remember, if you think you can, you will succeed. Think about the positive possibilities of losing weight steadily, easily, effectively, and effortlessly and you will lose weight.

If you are disagreeing with me at this moment about feeling positive with positive thoughts and saying to yourself that you have not achieved anything in your life, you would be very wrong! Do not be too quick to condemn yourself by finding faults with your behaviours or actions because you are perpetuating a negative pattern of behaviour which guarantees your failure in what you do.

Do not be too quick to argue and disagree with me because this is the basis of insecurity. Think about it seriously. If you have been quick to disagree with what I have said here it may be because there is anxiety in your life at the moment or because you have been using the word 'achieve' in a negative sense.

On the other hand, if you must doubt, ask yourself where your doubt is leading to. Would it help you to attain your goal of losing weight? Remember my point above that doubt is the opposite of believe. It dulls the edge of positive efforts and leaves your goal unfulfilled because doubt dampens positive effort.

Do not doubt yourself and your ability to succeed in achieving your goal. Look seriously and sincerely into your affairs and you will find that you have definitely achieved successes in your life. Take a deep breath, relax and look back with confidence and you will find plenty of successes in your life. Most important of all, remember that you have conquered some obstacles in life and got over certain difficulties in life to be where you are now.

In addition, you are now making plans for your success with the goal of losing weight steadily, easily, and effectively. You have started on this plan by reading this book and you will finish what you have started. You will finish it successfully because that is why you are reading this book, to achieve the success that you desire with your goal of losing weight.

Remember that this is a new method of losing weight that I am presenting to you. Remember the five fundamental principles that I discussed above and the secrets of how the human mind works. Remember your journey to the world of infinite positive possibilities. Remember that you are already a winner for making the journey successfully.

When you believe in yourself and think positive thoughts in the way that I am teaching you here, things will happen for you as you wish them to happen. They happen because you are making them happen by the effective use of the power within you.

Begin **today** to develop a different sense of value about yourself, self-worth, time, energy, work and your desire to lose weight. Begin from now onwards to evaluate yourself positively, to project a positive self image. Begin now to believe in yourself for this will help you to lose weight steadily, easily, effectively, and effortlessly. In this way, you will look good and feel great.

If you hold negative beliefs about yourself, about the idea of success in losing weight, then the thing to do now is to change your pattern of beliefs. Begin today to see that success is within your grasp because the magic power of success is within you. Start from now to believe in yourself and you will see an easy way out of any difficult situation.

Start from now to believe that there is **always** a way out of any problem. Begin now to do things differently from the way you have done in the past. This is what making a change is about. It is about doing something new or at least doing something in a different way from before. Start from today to believe that life is full of doors of opportunities opening up for you. Believe it for it is true. This book shows you how to do things differently from the way you have done them in the past. In following the instructions here and doing things differently from the way you had done them before, you are making a change to the existing situation because action is the route to change.

Use your mind positively to find a way out of any current problem which you may have. If you want to make progress in the face of mounting problems, remember to *always look on the bright side of life* and then do something new or, at least, different from what you have done in the past. As mentioned above, this book offers you something different, new methods of dealing with problems through mental action. Your mind is the womb through which all the fertile thoughts for positive mental constructions are incubated and hatched.

1.11 Key Points to Remember

- ❖ Remember that whenever you think positive thoughts about yourself, your goals and aspirations, you will find that positive feelings flow to you automatically.

- ❖ Always look on the bright side of life because irrational negativism dampens the spirits of positive action.
- ❖ Remember that belief is a detergent to doubt.

1.12 Positive Strategies to Enhance Your Success in Losing Weight
How to Guard Against Negatives in General

In order for an individual to achieve success in whatever venture he or she embarks on, he or she must endeavour to guard himself or herself against negative influences. Some negative influences may be of the individual's own making. Where this is the case, it is often difficult for the individual to recognise the negative influences upon him or her because people, in general, do not perceive themselves as impediments to their own progress.

Other negative influences may be the result of the activities of the negative people with whom an individual associates, that is, the company he or she keeps or the negative environment in which he or she works in or lives in. Whatever the negative feelings and negative thoughts an individual may have, and whatever the nature of those thoughts and feelings and how they may have been derived, the individual must be able to recognise the negative influences and eliminate them in order to feel mentally free to entertain positive thoughts about success.

This is particularly relevant in losing weight because your friends and associates may attempt to deter you from a chosen purpose by their negative vibrations. Stick to your plans and you will be successful in losing weight easily, steadily, effectively, and effortlessly.

An individual must become aware of his or her own will power and remember, always, that the magic of success is truly within him or her. The recognition of this will alert the person to the power of the unconscious mind and thus help him or her to eliminate negatives from his or her thoughts in relation to the goal of losing weight. An individual must become aware that negative thoughts will affect him or her if such thoughts are allowed to take hold in his or her unconscious mind.

In this respect it is most appropriate for an individual to avoid the association of people whose company drain the individual's energy psychically and makes the individual feel low, depressed or unhappy in some ways. If you wish to lose weight now, easily, steadily, and effortlessly you must avoid the association of negative people who constantly make you feel bad because of your weight and the way you look. It is not necessary to feel bad about yourself in order to lose weight. Feeling bad about oneself is negative feeling and this gives rise to self pity, low self esteem, lack of confidence and attendant anxieties associated with those negative feelings.

To eliminate the negatives influences of other people in an individual's life, the individual must master the five fundamental principles which I have discussed above because a sound knowledge of the five fundamental principles is a detergent to negative influences. An individual must also seek the company of people in whose association he or she gets an uplift, people who inspire him or her with confidence and make him or her feel good about himself or herself, or people whose achievements he or she admires and seeks to emulate.

1.13 Confront Your Fear to Conquer It

Do not be afraid of success because success is more desirable than failure. Some individuals are afraid to deal with the power, influence, and recognition that comes with the achievement of success but they convince themselves that they are afraid of failure. They are afraid of failure because they are thinking about failure so they fail to act on opportunities that come their way. Thus, they fail to accomplish their objective just as they fail to recognize their own negative thinking. Remember that if you are thinking too much about fear, this will be retained by your unconscious mind and, fear will become your reality.

Also, if you are thinking often about failure, the idea about failure will be imprinted on your unconscious mind. In this way, failure will become your reality and, it will be due to your thoughts. Do not be afraid of success. Do not think that you will fail because if you think of failure, failure will become your reality. Remember the fundamental principles discussed in this chapter. You must confront your fear and conquer it.

Fear is an impediment to your goal of losing weight and it can be manifested by your vacillation, procrastination, and doubting your own ability to succeed in losing weight. Sometimes people vacillate and procrastinate because they are uncertain of what to do and this uncertainty may be the result of insecurity which, also, leads to fear.

Thus, hear, there is a circle which can be a vicious circle in certain individual circumstances.

Fear is a hindrance to success in general and must be confronted for the individual to succeed in a chosen goal. Many sporting personalities and teams have lost competitions because they were afraid of the opponents or of the competition itself. Think about success in losing weight so that success will become your reality.

Fear is ordinarily an emotional or physiological response to a consciously recognized source of danger. The normal response takes the form of voluntary avoidance of the feared object. However, fear can occur unconsciously and may be employed by a person in a defence mechanism as a pretext to exculpate the failure to act in a certain way. Instances of such defences may occur if the person concerned has convinced himself or herself that he or she is afraid of attempting to lose weight because it will do damage to his or her body or to his or her looks.

In such circumstances, such a person, then, automatically avoids anything that will lead him or her to attempt to lose weight. Thus, he or she never takes part in any ventures to do with losing weight because of his or her fear of failure or fear of the alleged damage that losing weight may cause to his or her body or damage to the way he or she looks. The effect of such fear is that it destroys positive thoughts about losing weight, weakens the power of reflection on the advantages of losing weight and discourages positive effort in relation to losing weight and weight control in general.

Remember my discussions above about the powers of the unconscious mind. You will understand from this that fear will have a very dangerous effect on a person's attempt to lose weight. As I have described above, if a person is afraid of doing something, the natural response is to avoid the object or topic of fear. In doing so, the fear and its avoidance are retained in the unconscious. Thus, as the fear is retained in the unconscious, the individual perpetuates it automatically in motor activities. The individual becomes a very fearful and cowardly person.

Thus, when a person gives expression to fear in the form of negative and destructive thoughts about losing weight, he or she is very likely to experience the result of the fear in the form of destructive repercussions. The negative thoughts are retained in the unconscious and this becomes part of his or her general attitude, response, reaction, and behavioural traits in relation to losing weight. Such a person becomes a very negative, fearful, cowardly person lacking courage and moral fibre to make a definite decision to lose weight or to embark on anything worthwhile because of fear.

If a person wishes to lose weight and, at the same time, has fear of losing weight, fear that he or she might fail to lose weight, fear that his or her body may be damaged by losing weight then it is clear from my discussion of fear here, that such a person has a psychological conflict.

Such conflict is necessary in the development of neurotic anxiety and all those seemingly simple problems that blight an individual's enjoyment of everyday life. For a fuller discussion of **conflicts** in the development of psychoneurotic problems refer to my previous publication (Maurice-Nneke 2003).

Some anxiety problems may deter the success of lose weight programme. Anticipated traumatic stress disorder (**ATSD**) is an anxiety which is strengthened by negative thinking, insecurities, and self doubt. The individual has a morbid expectation that something will go wrong with a project or a venture. Thus, he or she avoids the venture or project because of the belief that it would go wrong. As applied to the project of losing weight the individual might feel strongly that something will go wrong with the plan to lose weight Now!

There is also **Murphy's Law,** a supposed natural law stating that anything that can go wrong will go wrong. This, like the anxiety above, is boosted by negative thinking, insecurities and self doubt. If you have a serious plan to lose weight, you must think positive thoughts about the success of your plan.

1.14 How to Deal With the Effects of Stress, Anxiety and Depression (SAD)

The effects of stress, anxiety, and psychological depression can be very damaging to a person's personality. They can lead to indolence, apathy, lack of confidence and very low self-esteem. Thus stress, anxiety and psychological depression bring about destructive negative attitudes which are barriers to progress in a chosen goal such as losing weight. Indeed, with some individuals stress, anxiety and psychological depression may be the cause of weight gain.

The people who suffer from anxiety problems, those who live or work in stressful environment or those who suffer from psychological depression, find it difficult to live in a healthy way. They may eat constantly for comfort and thus may put on weight heavily.

I use the term *psychological depression* to refer to an emotional problem of interpersonal relations which leads to a deep feeling of unhappiness and total inadequacy. This is distinguished from *organic depression* which is the result of some injury to the brain.

The unhappiness involved in psychological depression is often manifested in the individual's need to resort to food, alcohol or cigarette as a means of comfort, but it is in reality a means of escape for the individual, that is, the individual is running away from the need to confront the problem.

For some other people suffering from stress, anxiety and psychological depression, food, alcohol and cigarettes offer a means of denial of their problem by acting as a defence mechanism since for such people, the enjoyment of food, alcohol and cigarettes give the illusory feeling that everything is fine with them. Some people can put on a lot of weight by eating constantly for comfort.

A person who suffers from psychological depression has certain underlying psychological problems which make him or her feel very low and unhappy. As I have mentioned above, where certain underlying feeling of unhappiness exists in an individual's life, it is often difficult for the individual to attend positively to a goal such as losing weight.

Such a person, usually, resorts to negative attitudes such as self-pity, excuses and so on. Stress, anxiety and psychological depression are barriers to losing weight because they prevent an individual from concentrating fully on the tasks and exercises that are conducive to the goal of losing weight steadily, easily, effectively, and effortlessly. The apathy and lack of effort that results from inactivity prevents the person from looking good and feeling great.

To find out whether you are properly attuned in your mind to the goal of losing weight steadily, easily, and effectively, you must examine your private life thoroughly and answer the following questions truthfully and honestly to yourself.

- Do you have stress and anxiety in your life?
- Do you suffer from episodes of depression in your life?
- Are you depressed now?
- Are you prone to destructive negative thoughts most of the time?
- Do you live with people or a person who abuse you, bully or beat you?
- Do you eat often to comfort yourself?
- Are there people in your life who tell you that you are not good for anything?

Do not be troubled because it is not an intelligent test or an aptitude test. However, if you are frank and sincere in your answers you will find out more about your own personal issues and then be able to make improvements as necessary. If you admit to anxiety and depression, it is best that you deal with these problems first by consulting your own physician who may be able to recommend a psychotherapist.

You will find that the solution of the problems will enable you to concentrate more on your chosen venture of losing weight steadily, easily, effectively, and effortlessly. Here are the rest of the exercises which you must now administer to yourself before we proceed to the exercises for losing weight.

1.15 Examining Your Level of Stress, Anxiety, and Depression

Recognising the SAD Effect

A person who is afflicted with stress, anxiety, and depression is very usually a sad person. The sadness is often manifested in the behaviour or attitudes of the person. This can be noticed by other people such as family, friends or working colleagues with whom the sad person comes into contact. By coincidence the first letters of each of the words, *stress, anxiety, depression,* spell out **SAD** just as in the case of the condition known as *seasonal affective disorder.*

Stress leads to tension which conflicts with the existing situation and makes the individual to be unease, that is dis-eased. Thus, the individual has an illness. This is shown by the anxiety and depression which are treatable illnesses. Now you see the connections, if you do not know about them already. Find out whether the **SAD** effect is part of your personal issue or whether it is implicated in your behaviour or in your everyday attitudes towards people or things and events around you.

Answer the following questions in your own way but truthfully to yourself. If you choose to answer just 'YES' or 'NO' to any of the questions, let your 'YES' or 'NO' be represented by what happens to you most of the time with the situation described in the particular question. Do not say, 'It depends on...' This is not an answer to any of the question because we are dealing with general situations, not contextual or particular circumstances or isolated situations in your life.

However, if you choose to answer 'YES' or 'NO' to any question, be particularly careful that you do not answer 'YES' and 'NO' to the same question. For example, in the third question below, if your general attitude is to interrupt when people talk with you, then your answer to the question would be 'YES'. If you are unable to decide what your answer to a particular question should be and if you think that the questions have been cleverly but, intrusively designed to annoy, provoke, and force you to reveal your deep secrets, this is indicative that there are, indeed, certain underlying problems in your life.

If any of the questions make you say to yourself, "Everyone does that", you will be wrong because you do not **know** *everyone* however much you may wish to think that you do! At the best, all the people you know may be doing that but, all the people you know are not, strictly speaking, *everyone.* They are just *some* people that do whatever is implied in the question.

By saying to yourself or to others that "Everyone does that" you are, unconsciously, employing the psychological defence mechanism of *rationalisation.* You are trying to make your unwanted behaviour or habit 'fit' with what you think everyone does. This is to show that all is well with you, that you are the same as everyone else since your habit, action or behaviour is in accord with public habit, action or behaviour. However, you are not the same as everyone else and, you do not know everyone else.

By your rationalisation, you are defending yourself already before anyone has accused you of anything! When you are relaxed and keep your mind focused on deep relaxation with the methods which I show you in this book, you will find that everyone does not do whatever is implied in the questions.

Just relax and allow your mind to settle down and remember that your name does not appear anywhere on the questions. They are general questions and you are reading them alone in your own privacy and giving the answers to yourself. There is, therefore, nothing to be alarmed about.

Now, read carefully and answer all the questions sincerely and honestly to yourself in your own way. In order to determine the roots of SAD, if any, in your life you need to be truthful, honest and sincere to yourself in your answers to the questions.

1.16 Examining the Level of Anxiety in Your Life
1. In general, are you a negative or a positive person?
2. Would you describe yourself as an optimist or a pessimist?
3. Do you often interrupt when someone is talking to you?

4. *Are you always in a rush but really not accomplishing anything?*
5. *Can you wait your turn patiently in a queue?*
6. *Do you usually hide your feelings?*
7. *Do you do lots of things at once?*
8. *Would you describe yourself as a difficult person?*
9. *Do you often feel the need to cry no matter where you are?*
10. *Do you bite your nails from time to time?*
11. *Do you have any nervous twitches?*
12. *Do you find it hard to concentrate or make decisions?*
13. *Do you often feel irritable, snappy, or unfriendly?*
14. *Do you often find yourself eating when you are not hungry?*
15. *Do you regularly drink or smoke to calm your nerves?*
16. *Do you usually have a bad sleep at night?*
17. *Have you lost interest in sexual activities?*
18. *Do you feel always moody and distrustful of the people around you?*
19. *Do you blush when people look straight at you?*
20. *Are you a calm person who is not easily upset?*
21. *Can you sit still without fidgeting?*
22. *Can you keep your cool when your plans fail to work?*
23. *Are you afraid of the dark?*
24. *Does the thought of death, cancer, blood or heights bother you?*
25. *Have you ever used tranquillisers to calm your nerves?*
26. *Are you on tranquillisers now?*
27. *Do you think it is important to make an impression by your actions?*
28. *Do you examine your motives for the actions which you perform?*
29. *Are you bothered by what other people might be thinking and saying about you?*
30. *Do you think that you have bad luck and that other people are luckier than you?*
31. *Do you feel usually depressed when you wake up in the morning?*
32. *In general are you satisfied with the way things have turned out in your life to this moment?*
33. *Do you often suffer from loneliness?*
34. *Do you consider your future as quite bright?*
35. *Do you usually wake up in the morning with bad temper?*

36. Do you usually make hm, hm, hm, noises in apparent agreement but disinterestedly when someone is talking to you?

37. Do you usually create fictitious lovers and partners and tell lurid stories about your encounters with them in order to be popular with your peers and impress other people and make believe that you have a great social life and great sex life?

1.17 Examining Whether You are in Control

1. Are there some habits of yours that you would like to break but cannot?

2. Do you make your decisions in spite of what the people it concerns have to say?

3. If your plans fail to work do you usually accept responsibility for their failure or do you usually explain the failure away in ways that clears you of any blame?

4. Do you regularly feel that you are like a puppet that is being controlled by higher authorities or forces beyond your control?

5. Are you always convinced to act on issues only by the statements of other people?

6. Do you believe that it is possible for a person to change his or her personality?

7. Do you think that you can do things as well as other people?

8. Do you think about success or failure most of the time?

9. Do you think of yourself as a failure from time to time?

10. Are there many things about yourself that you would like to change if you could?

11. Do you care about other people's criticisms of your personality or your actions?

12. Do you often think that other people are better liked than yourself?

13. Can you say with sincerity that you are unashamed of anything you have ever done?

14. Do you often set your aspirations low in order to avoid disappointments?

15. Do you try to do things immediately rather than put them off until later?

16. Do you always try to finish the things you start?

17. Do you always tend to be jealous or envious of the success of other people?

18. Have you ever felt so angry that you would really like to kill someone?

19. If someone does you a bad turn do you usually ignore it?

20. Do you sometimes get so angry that you vandalize a property, break things or throw things around the house?

21. Do you usually have recourse to hysterical outbursts as your only course of action for attracting the attention of other people?

1.18 Examining Your Power to Project Yourself Positively

1. Do you usually seek revenge when someone hurts you in any way?

2. Would you rather agree with what someone had said so as to avoid an argument?

3. Do you feel that if someone is rude to you it is best to ignore them and let the occasion pass?

4. Do you often make sarcastic remarks about other people in their presence or behind their back?

5. Do you tolerate negative or discouraging influences around you which you can easily avoid?

6. If you have been waiting in a queue for a long time and someone came in and went straight to the front of the queue would you do something about it?

7. Do you usually put yourself second in matters relating to your family?

8. Do you believe that because of the way things are now it is necessary to fight for your rights or else you lose them completely?

9. Do you complain if an object which you purchased in good faith turns out to be an imitation?

10. If you were ignored in a public place such as in a restaurant, a meeting, a conference, a party, would you do something to get noticed or would you just disappear from the scene as quickly as possible?

If you have read the above questions carefully, and attentively, you would have noticed that I have touched on the issues raised by some of the questions in my discussions so far in this chapter. More of them would be touched on in the following chapters. Notice, also, that there are no scores for the questions.

The objective is for you to learn something about yourself. The questions provoke you into the examination of your motives and intentions for your behaviours, attitudes and actions in certain situations in your life. The questions above are the sort of questions which you will not, normally, ask yourself.

In giving serious attention to the above questions you will be delving deeper into the depth of the feelings that give rise to your actions in particular situations as implied in each question. In this way you will be able to make necessary changes to your life as required and you will have a clear, relaxed, frame of mind to focus on your goal of losing weight, and achieve the success that you desire.

1.19 Key Points to Remember

- ❖ Always guard against negative thoughts and endeavour to be positive at all times or as often as possible.
- ❖ Endeavour to eliminate the SAD effect, if any, from your life.
- ❖ Take control of your life and project yourself positively.
- ❖ The SAD effect in a person's life may cause that person to overeat and gain weight. In this way the person uses food as an oral gratification for the SAD symptom or their trigger.
- ❖ The SAD effect is always a barrier to the goal of losing weight for the reason given in the point above.

CHAPTER TWO: THE GOAL AND A PLAN OF ACTION FOR LOSING WEIGHT

You will get what you want for what you want is what you get

A prime requisite for success is to determine accurate goals or objectives. This is accomplished by establishing what you regard as your major and minor goals. A major goal should be those long range objectives which you hope to achieve within a long period of time.

For example, say within three years, five years or ten years and so on. This can be illustrated by the expressed desire in the following statement if the individual's major goal in life is to acquire abundant wealth and prosperity. *By this time in five years from now I will be a billionaire!*

A minor goal should be the short term range of objectives which you seek to achieve this month, within the next three months or six months as the case may be. In certain cases there may be a series of minor goals leading to the fulfilment of a major goal. In our case, the goal to lose weight can be a major goal for an individual if attaining the desired weight involves a long term plan or if the attainment of the desired weight would bring a major change in the individual's life as a whole.

2.1 How to Formulate the Goal to Lose Weight

For the specific purpose here of losing weight, a well formulated goal must have the following characteristics.

1. The Goal must be specific and defined clearly
Every individual has a series of ambitions, desires, hopes, needs, wants, wishes. These, initially, are not goals but each one of your ambitions, desires, hopes, needs, wants, or wishes can become your major goal or minor goal as the case may be.

This happens from the moment the particular ambition, desire, hope, need, want, or wish is isolated from the rest and made the central focus of your mental and physical energy. This is the energy required for your mental and physical efforts to achieve the objective. Refer to the third principle discussed above in the first chapter of this book.

To isolate any objective and make it into a goal you must put your series of ambitions, desires, hopes, needs, wants, and wishes into a scale of relative preference and deal with the one that is most pressing, most urgent, or most easily attainable. You must deal with the economic consideration involved. For example, the most pressing and most urgent objective may not be the most easily achievable.

Something becomes a goal for you when, after all the work of consideration and deliberations in evaluating its merits and disadvantages, you have isolated it from the series of other ambitions, desires, needs, wants, or wishes and so on, which are open to you, and you now focus all your mental and physical energies towards achieving that thing.

For example in order to achieve the goal of losing weight easily and effortlessly, the individual has to focus his or her attention on the health and the natural wholeness of his or her body, the need to eat low calorie healthy food, the need for positive thoughts about himself or herself and his or her ability to succeed in the goal. He or she must have self belief. Remember that no one is ready for success in any goal unless he or she believes that he or she is capable of achieving success in the goal.

Defining your goal clearly means that it should be properly distinguished from your range of other interests, ambitions, desires, need, wants, and wishes. It also means that the road to the fulfilment of your goal must be clearly mapped out showing what you ought to do, the length of time you have set aside to do it, and how you are to do what you ought to do in order to achieve the goal. In other words, defining the goal entails part of the action plan to accomplish the goal. Refer to my discussions of the plans of action for losing weight below in this chapter.

2. The Goal must involve new Behaviour or new Activity and a Plan of Action
When a goal is clearly formulated the formulation will include the definition of what the goal entails, and the plan of action that would

bring the goal about. The execution of this plan must involve you in new behaviours, doing things which you have not done before or things which you are not doing at the moment, or doing things differently.

Thus in order to achieve the goal you must be actively involved in a new form of activity or behaviour. In order to lose weight easily and effortlessly you must start with a new course of action such as the regime of mental action which this book brings to you.

As I stated in the introductory chapter above, this book is a journey into a new world, a new way of doing things, a new method of approach to personal and social problems, an adventure for self development and self improvement. It shows you a positive way to make your goal of losing weight easily achievable.

3. The Goal must be Positive and Realistic

If your goals are positive they become easy for you to fulfil and you will fulfil them much quicker if they are realistic. Losing weight will be a positive goal for an individual in relation to their health, height and weight. Here is an illustration to make the point clearer.

Suppose that a woman is 4ft tall and 20 stones in weight. Now, baring genetic and hormonal problems, the goal of losing weight will be a positive goal for her. The same applies for a man of the same stature. Suppose, on the other hand, that a man is 6ft tall and 7stones in weight with poor health. Now, for this man, the goal of losing weight will be a very negative and unrealistic goal for him. The same applies for a woman of the same stature.

4. The Goal must be Available

If you have taken great care and thought to formulate and define your goal you will see, easily, that if the goal is within your reaches, it will be attainable effortlessly. At one of my *Self Help Workshops* a gentleman participant stated that his goal was to own a Rolls Royce car. As he had no savings and investments and was earning only £100 per week from his employment at the time you can see, quite clearly, that the stated goal was not available to him at the time.

There is every reason to say that, although the goal was a positive one in so far as it was forward looking, it was indeed an unrealistic goal in respect of his financial position at the time. It is obvious that in view of his financial position the desire (for it was only a desire for him at the time not a goal yet!) for a Rolls Royce car will take an awfully long time to be accomplished. Thus, his immediate goal would, more appropriately, be a change of employment to a higher wage structure.

The goal to lose weight can be an available goal to any individual in respect of the particulars of his or her health if he or she is in a fit and proper condition to participate fully in all the practical exercises in this book. Refer also to my illustration above in relation to positive and realistic goals.

5. The Goal must be Located Within the Individual's Environment
The goal must be within your own environment or situation. For example if a person's goal is to be Prime Minister it follows that in order to achieve the goal, he or she must be a politician or else he or she never gets to achieve such a goal in a democratic country.

What happens in countries which are not democratic, where anyone can buy their way into high office or just seize power by armed means, is exceptional rather than the norm for the achievement of political goal. I am not concerned here with some devious and, sometimes, violent routes to the achievement of any goal as they are, for the purpose of this book, negative in so far as they cause harm and, perhaps, death to other people.

As in my illustration above, to be Prime Minister of a democratic nation like the United Kingdom, for instance, a person must be in politics and win his or her seat in a general election. He or she must also be the leader of the party that won the general election or be the winner of a party leadership contest by challenging the incumbent Prime Minister directly, or the winner of a leadership election in the event of a resignation or death of a Prime Minister.

What is relevant from these illustrations is that being a politician in a democratic country places the individual in a situation from which he or she can fulfil a goal of being Prime Minister. However, a British politician whose goal is to be the President of China, for example, would be setting his or her goal far beyond his or her environment and would be contending with different national culture and different political system thus making it too difficult or relatively impossible to fulfil the goal.

We would say from the above illustrations that the goal to lose weight is ordinarily within the environment of any individual since losing weight entails what one does to oneself. However, the method by which an individual chooses to do this might be stringent and thus, remote to the individual's metabolism.

The method which is advocated in this book is mental and so it is within the environment of every individual who is capable of thinking positive thoughts.

6. The Goal must be kept constantly in Mind
Remember from what I said above about the unconscious mind that your ideas must be clearly imprinted and fully developed in your mind for them to work for you. When you have taken the time and mental energy to formulate your goal, define it clearly and make a plan of action, it becomes necessary that you must keep the goal constantly in your mind in order to fulfil it.

It is quite obvious that failure to keep the goal constantly in your mind may make the goal more vulnerable to be forgotten completely or being replaced with other desires on your scale of preference. The goal to lose weight in the method which I am introducing to you here, is a goal of mental action so this is much more amenable to be kept in the mind.

2.2 How to Define Your Goal

Your goal must be stated clearly and precisely. One needs to be very specific in defining a goal. This is very important so that the action plans for achieving the goal are specifically directed and the mind is clearly focused on a particular goal. Your knowledge of the functions of the unconscious mind which I discussed above will help you to understand the need to be clear and specific in your definition of the goal.

The ultimate aim here is to attain the weight that you have chosen for yourself, the weight that you wish to be by time 'T' by losing weight steadily, easily, effectively, and effortlessly. Time 'T' is your signifier. It represents whatever element of time you wish it to represent in order to underline the urgency of your goal. You can state the goal in the following terms and this will also form part of your relaxation exercise. I shall write this out for your in the first person. In this way the goal will be firmly established in your mind.

My goal is to lose weight completely, to do so easily, steadily, effectively and effortlessly until I reach the weight that I have chosen for myself, the weight that I wish to be and to maintain that weight from this moment onwards. Losing weight steadily, easily, effectively and effortlessly will fill me with pleasure and happiness. I will feel the sensation of pleasure as the extra weight begins to drop off my body day by day in every way.

I will regard each weight that drops off my body as a sign of the success of my action plan and I will be very happy knowing that as each weight drops of my body day by day in every way, I am getting closer and closer to attaining the weight which I have chosen for myself, the weight that I wish to be. When I attain this weight I will be extremely pleased by what I have accomplished.

From that moment onwards I will become more and more conscious of my health. I will remember the essential health reasons that made it necessary for me to go on the journey to the world of infinite positive possibilities. Those reasons will be constantly in my mind with regard to eating. As a result of this, I will be eating for health and for the natural wholeness of my body.

From this moment onwards, I will be totally relaxed and completely in control because I know that I am achieving success with my goal. As I continue to be relaxed everyday and continue to lose weight, easily, steadily, effectively and effortlessly, I will find that the feeling of total relaxation, the feeling of being in control, the feeling of peace of mind and general well-being will stay with me and become part of my everyday feelings from this moment onwards. As I continue to be relaxed, I will look good and feel great day by day in every way.

As the feeling of relaxation increases in my life, I will notice that I am feeling very light and weightless, as light and weightless as if I can float way. This feeling of weightlessness increases my confidence and makes me more positive and optimistic in my outlook and I will love myself because of the success I am achieving with my goal. From this moment onwards as I continue to feel positive and happy, I will be able to show a positive mental attitude in anything I do and an attitude of love towards the people that matter in my life.

The above is the goal defined clearly in an unambiguous terms. It is important that the goal must be stated clearly and distinctly so that the unconscious mind understands your intention in relation to your goal of losing weight (or for whatever purpose). If the above definition of your goal is chosen it indicates to the unconscious mind that your chosen goal is to lose weight steadily, easily, effectively and effortlessly as I stated above.

2.3 Gaining Access to the Unconscious mind through Deep Relaxation

Now that your goal has been defined clearly, you must induce yourself into a state of deep relaxation in order to gain access to the unconscious mind. Why is it important to gain access to the unconscious mind? It is because that is where your ideas and mental prompts need to be imprinted for it to become part of your everyday motor actions. Ideas, mental prompts and other information received in the unconscious at moments of ultimate deep relaxation stay in the unconscious and influence behaviour.

As you will recall from my discussions in chapter one, the unconscious is not critical, judgemental or analytical like the conscious mind. The unconscious reproduces information faithfully like a tape recorder. You get out exactly what you have recorded. The objective here is always to record exactly what you want so that what you want will become your reality. With this objective in mind, you must begin with the following procedure.

2.4 How to induce yourself into a state of Deep Relaxation

Settle down and make yourself comfortable on a chair, couch or on the floor. Now, breathe in deeply, long and slow, through your diaphragm. Hold your breath to a mental count of five, or ten (or whatever number is suitable for you), exhale gently and allow the air to spread through your body as you R E L A X. Repeat this three or four times (or as many times as it is possible to loosen yourself up).

Now imagine yourself out in the open air. Make it a beautiful place and a beautiful day just as you would like it to be. You may choose to be on a sandy beach, in a park or even in your back garden. Wherever it is that you've chosen to be at this moment in your mind, make it a place which represents for you the very ultimate in peace, joy and total relaxation.

As you continue to relax this way from day to day you will find that you will feel very peaceful with each and every passing day. This feeling of peace and total relaxation will become a part of the way you feel from day to day. This feeling will become an attitude of mind and body for you. You will be very profoundly relaxed in mind and body wherever you happen to be and whatever the situation or the circumstances in which you find yourself, you will be absolutely relaxed and in control come what may.

Relaxation will give you the peace of mind and the inner tranquillity which will enable you to deal with the stress, the tensions, the worries and the anxieties that may intrude in your enjoyment of everyday life. You will be relaxed in mind and body and this will help you to take control of your life.

Now allow the feeling of relaxation to surge through every part of your body more and more. Begin from the top of your head and feel your scalp and your forehead relaxing, feel the muscles around your eyes relax, feel your cheeks and the muscles around your mouth relax, feel the whole of your face relax.

This feeling of relaxation begins now to spread down from your face to your neck and throat and from there it spreads across your shoulders and from your shoulders through your arms to the tips of your fingers with your wrists and your elbows very deeply relaxed. Concentrate now on your chest and your upper back and feel relaxation spreading from your chest to your abdomen and from your upper back to your lower back so that the trunk of your body is very deeply relaxed.

Now feel your waist and your bottom relax. This feeling of relaxation spreads to your pelvis, then it spreads down to your thighs, and from your thighs it spreads all the way through your knees and your lower legs to the tips of your toes. Your entire body is now going deeper and deeper into relaxation. Now I want you to feel it as relaxation surges through your body from the top of your head all the way down to the tips of your toes and from the tips of your toes it surges upwards to the top of your head. Feel it now as your entire body relaxes deeper and deeper.

As you continue to relax this way, you will find that the stress and the strain of the day will go out of your mind and out of your body. With increased relaxation you are able to let go your worries and your anxieties and allow the feeling of peace and inner calmness into your body and into your life.

You are now feeling a deep, profound relaxation in every part of your body. Your entire body is now deeply relaxed and serene. With this relaxation you should feel peaceful and comfortable.

As you become totally relaxed and completely in control, you may experience either a tingling sensation spreading through your body, or a feeling of elation or a feeling of lightness or weightlessness, as light and weightless as if you can just float away from where you are now. It is quite in order and proper to have any of those feelings or you may have a combination of those feelings for this indicates that you are totally relaxed.

As you are now deeply relaxed your unconscious mind is ready to receive positive instructions for your present and future well-being, for your happiness and to enable you to lose weight steadily, easily and effectively. You will be able to do so effortlessly because you will be relaxed always.

Note

As you are now deeply relaxed, your unconscious mind is now ready to receive positive instructions or mental prompts for your present and future well-being, for your happiness and to enable you to lose weight, steadily, easily, effectively and effortlessly. This note can also be incorporated in your relaxation technique as I have done it above thus allowing your goal of losing weight now, steadily, easily, effectively and effortlessly to be imprinted on your unconscious mind and become easily achievable by you.

The effect of this will be lasting for you because as your goal is imprinted in your unconscious mind your motor activities will reflect it. In this way the actions which will lead to the fulfilment of your goal will become part of your everyday motor activities. Refer back to the points that I made at the beginning of the above relaxation exercise about the need to gain access to the unconscious mind and also to the fundamental principles which I discussed in chapter one.

2.5 Positive Instructions and Mental Prompts

When you have attained a deep level of relaxation you can then give yourself positive instructions in relation to your desired goal which you have previously defined. The mental prompts can include the essential details of your goal as defined above.

I have defined a goal for losing weight above (Refer to section 2.2). Now for further illustration for the purpose of further exercise to be practised diligently, I want you to suppose that you have another goal which is to eliminate pain from your body. To make the illustration more interesting suppose, further, that it is the elimination of pain during childbirth. Male readers may concentrate on any excruciating pain they may have or on the pain of arthritis. We may begin as follows.

From this moment onwards when you use the word R E L A X, you will immediately feel as relaxed, comfortable, and serene as you are now. The word R E L A X will mean complete calm, peace, confidence and total tranquillity in your entire being. When the contractions begin during the birth of your baby the word R E L A X will turn the contractions to pleasurable sensations within your body and you will feel calm and confident.

You will be serene and anaesthetised to the contractions while enjoying happy, pleasurable, sensations in your body. These pleasurable sensations are a sign that your baby is about to arrive. The sign of the arrival of your baby fills you with great joy for you have waited for the arrival of your baby for a long time.

*As you are relaxed, you will be in total control throughout the birth because of your confidence and your knowledge that you have the **inner power to switch off** any unwanted sensation in your body. You will be full of joy, full of energy and vitality. The contractions will give you a feeling of joy.*

You will feel joy in the knowledge that your baby is about to arrive and the contractions are necessary for the arrival of your baby. You will feel pleasure as your baby enters the birth canal and each movement in your body gives you a pleasurable sensation in the knowledge that the waiting is all over and your baby is about to emerge.

The feeling of calm and confidence, joy and happiness will continue for you well after the birth of your baby and you will be always relaxed and in control, calm, full of confidence and contentment, full of energy and vitality day by day in every way. The birth of your baby will be a satisfying, pleasurable experience. You will feel totally relaxed and confident and you will show great love and affection for your baby and exhibit a positive attitude of love towards all your dear ones.

However, you do not need to be an expectant mother to apply the above relaxation technique for the control of pain. You can use the above technique to control pain in other areas of your body where excruciating pain is felt such as the pain of arthritis, cramp, rheumatism, backache, migraine and so on. Female readers may use the technique to control period pains. For more relaxation exercises relating to the control of pain during childbirth, refer to chapter one of my book previous book (Maurice-Nneke 2002).

Note

Notice, that I have used some of the positive expressions that I used at the preparatory exercises in chapter one. This is for familiarity. Your mind is already familiar with these positive words and will react to them positively when you focus your mind clearly on your objective.

In this particular exercise, if you cannot remember the essential details of your goal, it is sufficient to use a summary that contains the gist of what you want to achieve. Always use positive expressions and avoid the use of negative terms at all times. Always affirm the things that you want to achieve, not their negation. Examine the following illustrations.

(A) *During the birth of my baby I will not panic, and I will not feel any pain.*
(B) *During the birth of my baby I will feel a pleasurable sensation in my body and I will feel calm, confident, totally relaxed and absolutely in control.*

Notice that (A) is a negative and dangerous affirmation while (B) is a positive affirmation or mental prompt. Always be on your guard against the temptation to make such negative, and dangerous affirmation as in (A) above.

As mentioned above, I have used the pain of childbirth here merely for the purpose of illustration. Male readers and other females who are not expectant mothers can use the pain of arthritis or any other physiological pain which they may have. Remember that the gist of the mental prompts in the illustration can be applied to the goal of losing weight, and feeling good generally.

The above procedure is what you need for your goal to lose weight. However, I shall show you more techniques in the next chapter so that you have the option to choose the most appropriate method for yourself.

2.6 Key Points to Remember
- ❖ It is necessary to be deeply relaxed in mind and body for the purpose of bringing about the desired changes.
- ❖ It is necessary to use positive words always for your mental prompts.

Now I want to show you how everything that I have said here about goals fits in with an individual's actual goal of losing weight. I shall do so by examining the problem of the individual.

2.7 Problem: The Alcoholic Chocolate Cake Lady
A young woman gave the following information about herself and her problems during her consultation. For the purpose of the illustration and my discussions here I designate the young woman as the *Chocolate Cake Lady.* Here is a condensed vignette of her problem.

I am 32 years old, 25 stones in weight. I am an avid eater of chocolate cakes and I overindulge on alcohol, drinking an average of about fifteen pints of bear and six bottles of wine a week. I also drink the hard stuff, whisky, vodka, brandy, gin, rum and others. I enjoy these pleasures enormously but unfortunately people stare at me in the pubs (public houses). I don't care, I drink alone.

My love life is zero. I do not have a man in my life and I cannot remember the last time, if ever, I had a man in my life. Men are not interested in me. They seem to run away from me. Some of them laugh at me. I think this is because I am grossly out of shape and awfully unattractive to men. It is not their fault.

I would really like it for a man to smile at me and fancy me instead of laugh at me but I don't see how this could happen. However, I cannot be bothered with them. I know that I do not care about how I look; my appearance, make up and all that do not interest me. I think it is all a waste of time. It's the way I am.

2.8 Weight Loss Goal: To Lose Weight by Time 'T'

I believe that the formula for the management of a successful lose weight programme would be to fit a clearly defined goal with a serious action plan. This could be stated as SLWP = CDG + SAP, where SLWP is *successful lose weight programme,* CDG is *clearly defined goal,* and SAP is *serious action plan.* An appropriate way of showing how the formula works will embrace the following procedures for setting the appropriate clearly defined goals.

Remember that I am talking to you here about **the power of the mind.** I am talking about how you can use the thinking power of your mind to achieve your goals successfully. It is, also, about how those who are negatively inclined can prevent themselves from achieving a desired success by their negative thoughts.

If you have followed my discussions here attentively, you would be able to see quite easily, clearly, the power of the young lady's negative thoughts. By using your mind solely for negative thoughts you would be eliminating yourself from the benefits of the opportunities around you and, thus, preventing yourself from achieving the success that you would, otherwise, have enjoyed, yet blaming your failure on other people!

In the lady's case her love of chocolate cakes, alcoholic tendencies, and negative thinking were preventing her from enjoying a desired romance. It is obvious that she yearns for a heterosexual romantic liaison because her problem is introduced to us as a *complaint.* This indicates that the current situation is an unwanted intrusion into her life, perhaps it is an intolerable situation.

However she puts a damper on any positive efforts on her own part by saying that men are not interested in her, they laugh at her and run away from her yet, at the same time, she yearns for a man to smile at her and fancy her! She tells us the reason why men are not interested in her is because she is out of shape and awfully unattractive to men.

Now in saying this she, unconsciously, plays the *self pity* card which, in this instance, is a defence mechanism against the idea of taking positive action to maintain her looks and appearance and present a generally attractive personality. This form of defence is known as *rationalisation.*

It sounds good on the surface but deep down it prevents the individual from taking positive action on any particular uncomfortable, or unwanted situation. The *Chocolate Cake Lady* takes her stated reason to be an affirmation of truth and so does nothing about it. She resigns herself to the existing situation which is a situation she does not want. Thus, here, there is a conflict which is usually the causal origin of psychoneurotic problems.

We can also view the *Chocolate Cake Lady's* problem in a simpler way in relation to the account which I have given here about the power of the unconscious mind. It is clear from her statements that the *Chocolate Cake Lady* is affirming what she does not want, that is, affirming the negation of what she really wants.

This is also laden with conflict and as a result of the things she has affirmed, she gets what she has affirmed because this is what has been imprinted on the unconscious mind. Her negative thinking provides her with an excuse for not bothering to take care of her general appearance. *There is always a way out of any problem* through the positive use of the powers of the mind.

Now, let us turn the *Chocolate Cake Lady's* desire for romance into a goal of losing weight with the incentive of obtaining a boyfriend and see how a positive frame of mind will help her to fulfil her desire. This positive frame of mind will be implicated in her beliefs, attitudes, the way she channels her energy and it is best described as an *action plan.*

2.9 How to Make an Action Plan for the Goal: To Lose Weight at time 'T'.

The fulfilment of any goal requires a positive frame of mind which is defined in an action plan. An *Action Plan* is a definite, serious plan of action, activities, or tasks which must be performed in order to accomplish the goal. It sets out the course of actions, sets out the various actions which are necessary for the fulfilment of the desired goal. For the stated goal on behalf of the *Chocolate Cake Lady,* the necessary actions and attitudes to achieve the goal must include the following.

2.10 Action Plan 1: Expressing Self Belief

- ❖ I can lose weight steadily, easily and effectively because I believe that I have the power to do so and I will do so effortlessly.
- ❖ I can lose weight steadily, easily and effectively because that is my goal.
- ❖ I can lose weight steadily, easily and effectively because I am concerned for my health.
- ❖ I believe that I am an attractive, charming woman with magnetic personality and men are irresistibly drawn to me.
- ❖ I believe that I am attractive to men because men are always interested in me and they smile at me always.
- ❖ I can get a boyfriend because I am an attractive and beautiful woman.
- ❖ I know what I want and how to get it.
- ❖ I am an approachable, sociable and loveable person.

2.11 Action Plan 2: Act with Positive belief and Show this in Attitudes about Romance

- ❖ I believe that I am a desirable woman because every woman is desirable.
- ❖ I am a beautiful woman and I care about my health and beauty.
- ❖ I take particular care about my appearance because I like to look good always.
- ❖ I will accomplish my goal by losing weight at time 'T'

2.12 Action Plan 3: Translating Action 2 into Positive Practical Action

- ❖ I care very much about looking good and feeling great always.
- ❖ I will always pay attention to my clothes and my personal hygiene.
- ❖ I will always pay attention to my overall appearance.

❖ I will refrain more and more from eating chocolate cakes.

❖ I will refrain more and more from the habit of overindulgence on alcohol and cut down on my intake of beer, wine and spirits.

❖ I will pay more attention to my overall physical appearance by doing exercises.

❖ I will practise the relaxation exercises outlined in this book.

❖ I will perform positive actions to lose weight steadily, easily, and effectively. I believe that I will do so effortlessly.

2.13 Action Plan 4: Be Confident in the Knowledge that You Are an Attractive Woman

❖ True knowledge of something entails knowing that one knows it. If one knows something this is easily manifested by making use of the knowledge constantly. The *Chocolate Cake Lady* must show that she knows that every woman is attractive, and that includes her. She must accept herself as an attractive lady so that others will accept her too. If you believe that you are an attractive woman, so be it that is what you are. The belief will help the *Chocolate Cake Lady* to make herself looking more attractive from day to day.

❖ The *Chocolate Cake Lady* must affirm the knowledge and belief which is expressed in action plans 1 and 2 by showing self confidence in her actions.

❖ The *Chocolate Cake Lady* must be positive about herself, by socialising with men. She must learn how to smile so that men can smile back at her.

❖ The *Chocolate Cake Lady* must endeavour to make use of the knowledge that she can lose weight now and that she can do so steadily, easily, effectively, and effortlessly! In this way she will look good and feel great.

❖ The *Chocolate Cake Lady* must perform all the activities which are amenable to the fulfilment of the goal.

❖ The *Chocolate Cake Lady* must make use of positive mental prompts to affirm her goal of losing weight, and keep that constantly in mind.

2.14 Action Plan 5: Affirming the Goal

* ❖ The *Chocolate Cake Lady* must keep the goal constantly in her mind through a general positive outlook on the possibility of its attainment.

* ❖ The *Chocolate Cake Lady* must **go for it** and lose weight now easily and effortlessly in order to win her man in the most subtle way using her, natural, feminine charm and allure. Any serious female can do this very well without going over the top.

* ❖ The *Chocolate Cake Lady* must remember not to sell herself short by being cheap and at the same time, not to over price herself by a pretentious superiority and aloofness. She must adopt a serious attitude towards the achievement of the goal.

* ❖ The general rule for the *Chocolate Cake Lady* is to remember her self-worth and think of herself as an attractive lady, a lovable lady (see action 1).

* ❖ The *Chocolate Cake Lady* must perform the preparatory exercises given in chapter one in order to actualize her goal.

In the name of honesty and sincerity, if the *Chocolate Cake Lady* is serious about losing weight, and having a relationship, she must not play silly games about being too hard to get. This does not imply that she should pair herself off with any Tom, Dick or Harry that comes along. On the contrary, it means, quite simply, that she must be serious about the fulfilment of the goal and endeavour, as necessary, to make compromises by relinquishing all indecisions about the 'real' man, the 'ideal' man or the 'type' of man she is looking for, whatever theses versions of man are meant to be.

By being indecisive about what she wants, she will get no one and thus, defeat the purpose of the goal. Remember the power of the unconscious mind and how it deals with vacillations, indecisions, and negative mental prompts. If your mental prompts are ambiguous, or if you are uncertain about what you want, the unconscious mind will record nothing for you because ambiguity and indecisions are not goals or wishes.

If you use negative mental prompts, the unconscious mind will record for you the opposite of what you really want. Since your intention is to achieve success with your goal, the reality will be failure on account of your negative mental prompts.

The *Chocolate Cake Lady* must remember from my discussions of the power of the *unconscious* in chapter one above, that when ideas which are not clear and distinct are recorded in the unconscious the result will be the negation of what the individual wants. In like manner, negative and confused thought bricks produce the negation of what the individual really wants because the unconscious is confused by them. Refer to my account of the unconscious mind in section 1.5 above.

In terms of social, or romantic, relationship some ladies feel coy about making the first approaches. Though this is a good attitude which indicates an individual's good upbringing, social and moral background, one should not allow such attitude to preclude one from enjoying a much desired relationship.

There are ways in which a lady can make compromises without undermining her principles or seeming to be forward. The individual must be positive and realistic and go with the circumstances of each event, or situation without seeming to fall below his, or her moral standard.

In short, any lady who is seriously seeking heterosexual relationship must not allow herself to be pretentiously prudish because, after all, this is a new millennium of female consciousness and liberation which is far different from the moral hypocrisy and pompous conservatism which was the hallmark of attitudes and behaviours over recent past centuries. If you are a woman, I hope that you understand what I mean, and I trust that you know what to do when the opportunity comes your way.

Notice that I have put a time element, time 'T' on the goal. It is this that transforms the *Chocolate Cake Lady's* desire for a romantic liaison into a goal for losing weight in order to find a boyfriend. The time element fixes the goal on her unconscious mind. The actions necessary to accomplish the goal have an additional effect of helping her to lose weight. The time element underlines the urgency of her desire to lose weight and helps her to keep it constantly in mind.

Notice, also, that the goal and the plans for its achievement involve the *Chocolate Cake Lady* in new activities and in positive thoughts which bring about positive feelings. I have used a young woman's complaint for my illustration. Depending on the context of a particular problem, the same procedures are also applicable for a man.

2.15 How to Acquire the Will to Succeed in Losing Weight

Remember that you must keep the goal alive in order to fulfil it. Refer to the five fundamental principles in chapter one and you will find that the more deeply you understand the importance of the above factors, the more effectively you will be able to apply them in your daily life.

In this way, you will be successful in whatever undertaking you embark on and you will certainly be successful in losing weight easily, and effortlessly. In this way you will look good and feel great always. If you put your mind seriously into achieving success in losing weight, you must go for it so that you lose weight now!

Use your mind positively. Give up all restrictive negative attitudes and propel yourself to success because it is clear that out of the world of any endeavour, success begins with an individual's will to succeed. In every endeavour that you embark on, negative thoughts are the things that are most likely to prevent you from achieving the success that you desire.

Most important of all, you must always bear in mind the five fundamental principles of mind power which I have discussed in the first chapter of this book. Remember that the thought bricks for success or failure are constructed in the mind and always endeavour to construct the bricks for success. Try to understand and master the following little verse which clearly underlines the five fundamental principles of mind power which I discussed in chapter one of this book.

If you think you are beaten, you are.
If you think you dare not, you don't.
If you like to win, but think you can't,
It is a cinch you won't win.

If you think you will lose, you have lost.
For out of the world we find,
Success begins with a fellows will,
It is all in the state of mind.
If you think you are outclassed, you are.
You've got to think high to rise,

You've got to be sure of yourself before
You can ever win a prize.
Life's battles don't always go
To the stronger or faster man,
But soon or late the man who wins
Is the man who thinks he can.
(Anonymous)

In any situation, if you think you can, you are already on your way to the winning post. It is all in the state of the mind. Success begins in the mind. This is the essence of mind power. Thus, with your lose weight programme, you must always attune your mind to success and you will be for ever successful.

Remember that *the magic of success is within you.* It is within your mind. Apply the magic now in everything that you do from day to day starting from today and you will find that you can lose weight now! You can do so steadily, easily, effectively, and effortlessly by adhering to all the principles in this book, the principles of rational, positive action.

CHAPTER THREE: LOSING WEIGHT STEADILY, EASILY AND EFFECTIVELY

If you have built castles in the air, your work need not be lost: that is where they should be. Now put the foundations under them (Henry David Thoreau, 1817 - 1867).

3.1 Deep Relaxation as Weapon for Losing Weight

I have discussed deep relaxation for the goal of losing weight in the last chapter. In this chapter I offer you other ways of arriving at deep relaxation for the same purpose. Now you have a choice of what methods to adopt. The procedure, that is the steps to follow, is the same but the scripts, imagery and pictorial representation are different.

Always remember that deep relaxation is an indispensable aid to losing weight through the practical mind technique as it helps the individual to stay focused on the chosen objectives. In order to lose weight steadily, easily and effectively one must, first, learn how to attain a profound level of relaxation both mentally, and physically.

By following this method, you will be able to lose weight steadily, easily, effectively and do so effortlessly. In this way, you will feel good and look great always. With practice, you will be able to attain your own required level of deep relaxation within minutes or seconds of your trying. It is that simple and I am going to show it to you here again, right now, as I did in the last chapter. As the saying goes, *the taste of the pudding is in the eating.*

Surprisingly enough, most things within the field of depth psychology bear truth to the above saying. The techniques in the practice of depth psychology are much better understood after an individual has been through it via therapeutic analysis for self knowledge in the nature of finding out more about his or her inner self. In like manner, in the particular case of losing weight, an individual can focus much deeper on a chosen objective when he or she is deeply relaxed or when he or she has developed a relaxed attitude as a way of life.

I am dealing here with very practical personal affairs and the best method of approach in the application of practical matters is to practise by using the method that you want to understand or learn about. With depth psychology one does not need to be ill or emotionally unbalanced in order to learn to understand one's inner self.

The questions which I asked you in chapter one to test the SAD effect in your life are truly exploratory questions which will help any serious reader to acquire self knowledge as those questions relate to purely personal issues which may be deep rooted issues for some individuals.

Before the experience of self knowledge some people are usually ignorant objectors and a few may be uncritical apologists. As I mentioned, also, in chapter one, with ESP powers it is always better to have an open mind. Allow yourself the freedom to embark on the road of exploration as I also invite you to do with the preparatory exercise in chapter one.

3.2 Practice Session – The Relaxation Techniques

In order to practice how to focus the mind on the idea of losing weight steadily, easily, effectively, and effortlessly, you will need to proceed with a method of deep relaxation as follows.

1. Breathing Exercise

Firstly, find a comfortable position either sitting on a chair or lying on a couch or on a bed, or on the floor if that is more comfortable for you. Now take a long, slow deep breath through your diaphragm. Hold your breath for a mental count of about five, or ten, or twenty, or whatever number is comfortable for you before you run out of breath. Choose the length of hold to suit your desired level of relaxation.

Then, open your mouth slightly, and slowly exhale as you allow the air out of your body and let go all negative thoughts as the air leaves your body and let go, let go, let go, let go, let go as you drift deeper, deeper, and deeper, into relaxation, allowing the feeling of peace and total relaxation to spread from the top of your head all the way down to your toes. Repeat the process three times.

This means that you will be performing four breathing exercises in all. If you have done this properly, diligently, as you read these lines, you should feel the sensation of relaxation moving through your body, now. Your body should now feel all loosened up.

However, if you don't feel loosened up at this stage it is because you are tense, nervous or fighting with yourself in being sceptical, doubting your own ability to do it well. If this is the case, don't worry. I tell you that you can do it; it is really very simple. Remember that you can do it because you have done it before in every previous chapter right from your journey to the world of infinite positive possibilities in the preparatory exercise in chapter one. You also did it in chapter two in relation to your goals and mental prompts. Now, relax and let go your negative thoughts and negative feelings, if any, and repeat the procedure until you feel loosened up. Start now.

There is no fixed rule on how many times you have to repeat the procedure. Many people feel at ease after one deep breathing exercise and some other people need to repeat the exercise a few times in order to feel at ease. Do what suits you the best, but do the exercise. Do not skip it over because it is a necessary part of the practice of losing weight with the practical mind technique which I introduce to you in this book.

You will recall that at the end of the preparatory exercise in chapter one, I told you that if you are able to perform the preparatory exercise diligently, and successfully, all other exercises in this book will become easy and great fun for you. This is the time to put all your learning into practice. Remember, also, the five fundamental principles above and try to think more about the great power of your mind and your ability to succeed in what you aim to achieve.

If you believe truly, that you can do it, you will. Always read the verse at the end of chapter two to encourage you and give you a confidence boost. However, if you feel any discomfort while doing the exercises, you must discontinue immediately and wait until you feel comfortable enough to continue.

2. Deep Relaxation Exercise

When you have completed the breathing exercises, your next move is to relax every part of your body by focusing your thought or concentrating your attention on each particular part of your body that you wish to relax.

When you have mastered this technique of deep relaxation, you will find that at any time you direct your thoughts to any part of your body and say to that part (or command it) to *r e l a x,* it will obey your command, immediately. It will begin to relax and you will start to feel at ease straight away.

This might sound implausible to you at first but with practise you will be able to prove it for yourself. When this happens, you will be in control at any moment of tension, or crisis, and in any situation. Remember, that whenever you use your mind to say to yourself, *r e l a x,* or shout the word out if necessary, you will feel relaxed instantly, and you will be able to take control of the situation.

In practising the techniques for losing weight, you will be speaking directly to your unconscious mind. Since I have already discussed the power of the unconscious mind and how it records the data of your life, you can see now how you can lose weight steadily, easily, and effectively by recording your goals about losing weight directly in your unconscious mind as I did in the last chapter.

This is part of the power of your unconscious mind. It has the power to record information. You will be instructing your mind to do what you want, in this case, to effect deep relaxation in your life. In this way you will be able to relax easily but, overall, the action plans for your goal will be manifested in your motor activity as you begin to perform, easily, effortlessly, all the everyday actions that are necessary to make your desired weight become a reality for you.

Note that it is also effective to speak directly to your unconscious mind in the second person. However, you may speak in the first person if you prefer. This is effective too. If this is what you want, you can adapt all the texts which I have given here in this book in order to enable you to speak in the first person. You can now begin to speak to your unconscious mind by telling it to effect deep relaxation in your body. You may begin in the following way.

You are now entering a state of deep relaxation. Your feet are becoming more and more deeply relaxed. This feeling of relaxation is spreading upwards from the tips of your toes through your feet to your ankles, legs, knees and thighs. Your limbs are getting more and more relaxed.

The feeling of relaxation increases from your thighs and spreads to your bottom, your waist and your pelvis. This feeling of deep relaxation is slowly spreading to your abdomen, your stomach, your chest, and your back. You are getting more and more progressively relaxed. Your entire body is becoming relaxed and you feel very light, weightless and absolutely serene as you are becoming deeply relaxed.

Now, shift your attention to your hands as this feeling of serenity is spreading to all parts of your body. Your hands are becoming very deeply relaxed. The feeling of serenity and deep relaxation continues to flow upwards through your body from the tips of your fingers through your wrists, your hands, your elbows, your arms, all the way up to your shoulders.

Now as you are feeling relaxed, this feeling of relaxation surges across your shoulders so that your shoulders are deeply relaxed, very deeply relaxed. You now feel peace and tranquillity flowing through your whole body from all directions.

The feeling of relaxation continues to surge from your shoulders upwards to your neck and throat, and then across your face and up to the top of your head. Your scalp, your forehead, your cheeks, and your jaw are all very deeply relaxed. You are now experiencing a very profound feeling of relaxation in every part of your entire body.

The whole of your body is deeply relaxed, peaceful, and comfortable. Your mind is calm, very quiet and tranquil. You are now perfectly in tune to give further information about losing weight to your unconscious mind. The information which you give will become part of your motor activity from now onwards and it will help you to lose weight steadily, easily, effectively, and you will do so effortlessly.

Notice, that steps 1 and 2 above are known as *Induction*. In my discussion in the previous chapter, I have described this as '*Inducing yourself into a state of Deep Relaxation*'. It is the same procedure but different way of arriving at deep relaxation. Do what suits you best.

3. The Instruction or Mental Prompts

You have now arrived at the crucial point at which to give dynamic instructions or mental prompts to your unconscious mind in order for your unconscious mind to produce the desired effect for you from now onwards. In the next section I shall deal with how to give this information to your unconscious mind.

Basically what I am saying is that when you have completed the breathing and the relaxation exercises correctly, you should be in the ideal frame of mind and disposition to give instructions or mental prompts to your unconscious mind to effect the changes which you require in your life at any particular moment.

In this instance what you need is to speak to the unconscious mind about losing weight steadily, easily, effectively and about being able to do so effortlessly. You must be serious about what you say and mean what you say.

Always remember the five fundamental principles which I discussed in chapter one of this book. The thoughts that you have most often in your mind will become your reality. If your unconscious mind is fed constantly with the weight that you have chosen for yourself, the weight that you wish to be, this will become your reality and you will lose weight steadily, easily, effectively and effortlessly because eating low calorie healthy food will become part of your everyday motor actions. You just do it easily, naturally, effortlessly because your unconscious mind has got the message.

It is that simple but you will have to be serious about it for it to happen. You have to be specific about your intentions and speak to the unconscious mind in unambiguous terms. Remember that the unconscious mind reproduces things exactly as you have presented them, just like a tape recorder. It is also important that you believe, wholly and firmly, in what you are saying to the unconscious mind and not merely verbalise it parrot fashion.

3.3 The Dynamics of Mental Prompts

Mental prompts are personal instructions or personal information which you give to your mind with the desire for the particular instruction or information to become your reality. The practical mind technique which I present to you in this book gives you the simplest method of recording information in the unconscious mind.

Remember that anything recorded in this way remains in the depth of unconsciousness but is at the same time very active as it affects an individual's motor actions. Everything that you say to the unconscious mind in a deep state of relaxation remains in the unconscious but is manifested in your everyday motor actions. If you have forgotten about this you may now refer to my description of the power of the unconscious mind in chapter one.

Since your particular aim at the moment is to lose weight steadily, easily and effectively, the information which you give to the unconscious mind will reflect this aim in order to make your desired weight a reality. This method of recording information in the unconscious consists of personal instructions given by you to your unconscious mind thus facilitating instant replay of the required information in your everyday motor actions.

You start in a simple way by giving simple information or instructions to the unconscious mind. Initially this will serve the purpose of getting yourself into the routine of giving mental prompts to the unconscious mind for the things which you desire to surface in your life through your everyday actions.

As you become adept in the use of mental prompts, you will find that the sky is the limit for you, because you can use the prompts to achieve anything you wish to achieve, to deal with anything in which you seek to achieve success. Indeed, to get what you want.

As you become relaxed and focus your mind deeply on what you wish to achieve, you will speak to your unconscious mind seriously about what you want to achieve. Soon with your actions, you will find that what you desire becomes your reality. Deep relaxation is the key to the success of mental prompts.

The personal instruction, or personal information, which I describe as mental prompts are mental directives, ordering your unconscious mind to act on the information or instruction which you have given. Your unconscious mind acts on it to make your desire a reality. It works through your motor activities because your unconscious mind acts on any information it receives.

Thus the personal instructions, or personal information which you give to your unconscious mind must be direct, definite, simple and, preferably, given mentally. However, you may give your orders or instructions audibly if this is more convenient for you. In whatever form you may choose to give your mental prompts, you must take note that it is best to give the mental prompts during the moment of ultimate deep relaxation as mentioned above.

At this point of deepest relaxation you have established optimum conditions to give your mental prompts of personal instructions or personal information for your unconscious mind to receive them freely. This point of ultimate relaxation is the moment at which your mind is absolutely receptive and it is uncluttered by doubts and negative thoughts. You can see from this why it is more advisable to give the personal instructions or personal information mentally.

Whatever it is that you wish to accomplish in your life you can do so with the practical mind technique that I introduce to you in this book. To use the technique you will always make use of mental prompts but as I have mentioned above, it is always best to use the mental prompts technique of personal information or personal instruction immediately during the moment of ultimate relaxation.

If you have a lot of different instructions or information to give to your mind, you will find that it is very beneficial to put these in a sequence that is logical and meaningful to you. Take particular care in the knowledge that your unconscious mind accepts information as presented. If what you say is careless, meaningless or ambiguous, your desired reality will not materialise!

It is also important that your mental prompts which consist of the personal instructions or personal information that you give to your unconscious mind should be in your own words, words that, as mentioned above, are meaningful to you and tailored to each specific area, problem or situation in your life which you wish to confront. Always use positive words to do this. Do whatever suits your particular requirements and what works best for you.

Give your instructions or personal information and, then, allow the unconscious mind to work on it for it to happen. For example, after you have used the relaxation technique and you feel that you are in the moment of ultimate relaxation, you may let your first personal instruction be to direct your unconscious mind to accept the word *r e l a x* as your instant cue for relaxation.

You may give the instructions in the first person by changing the text for that purpose. I am giving the instruction to you here, so I have written the text in that way, but you can adapt it. The instructions to the unconscious can be given as follows.

From this moment onwards wherever you happen to be, whatever the occasion, whatever the circumstances, whomever you happen to be with, when you use the word 'r e l a x', you will become relaxed immediately, feeling comfortable and serene as you are now. The word 'r e l a x' will mean complete calm, peace, contentment and total relaxation in your life.

This is an excellent positive instruction at this stage because by it you are instructing your unconscious mind to make the feeling of relaxation a part of your life. What will happen with this suggestion is that the feeling of relaxation will become an attitude of mind and body for you and you will cease to feel tense, edgy, nervous or irritable. You will be relaxed in difficult situations, come what may, you will be in control, calm, relaxed in mind and body and totally unfazed by any situation or crisis.

The positive instruction which I have used above should be familiar to you. I used the same tones in the positive instruction given in the main preparatory exercise in chapter one above. The objective of the preparatory exercise at the time was to set the psychical system in motion and accustom your mind and body to the regime of deep relaxation.

Notice, also, that in the above instruction I said that "you will become relaxed immediately, feeling comfortable and serene as you are now".

This is to underline my previous suggestion that your instructions or mental prompts must be given to your unconscious at the moment of ultimate relaxation. They should be given always at the moment in your relaxation exercise when you attain ultimate relaxation and feel peaceful and serene.

The purpose of the instruction, therefore, is to allow your unconscious mind to save this moment for you and make it a permanent part of your life which you can playback or bring on at any time you use the word *r e l a x*. Remember this, always. This is why you can order it and receive it because it is there for you.

You may understand this better with reference to your computer files. When you save a file on your computer, you can open it up by clicking on the name of the file and it opens up for you again. Remember that the computer merely mimics what the human mind does naturally. Your mind is more prodigious than the most sophisticated computer because the computer is a creation of the human mind.

This act of giving simple instruction to your unconscious mind will bring about positive results in your life in whatever goal you wish to accomplish. It is important to distinguish the act of ordering, commanding or giving instructions to your mind from the act of giving suggestions.

The act of ordering, commanding or giving instructions to your unconscious mind involves you in making a positive demand from your unconscious mind, ordering it to do what you want. It is like placing an order for something. Remember also the powerful force of the positive instructions in the preparatory exercises at the beginning of chapter one.

In the above example, you are giving an order which is to be executed by your unconscious mind to the extent that each time you use the word *r e l a x,* you will feel, from that moment onwards, an automatic and instant relaxation in mind and body.

It will also bring about a highly desirable state of total calm whenever you desire it. It will do so wherever you happen to be. Whether you are travelling on a crowded train, whether you are taking an examination or having a job intervie. It will also happen when you are in a business meeting or, participating in competitive sports event or, driving a car. This technique will also help you to feel calm and relaxed in a busy traffic or in moments of minor personal crisis.

All you need to do in these situations is say the word *r e l a x* and you will feel relaxed, instantly. You can say the word mentally, whisper it or say it audibly as circumstances may require.

The same procedure applies in losing weight. Remember that you have to be specific when making mental prompts. You must be clear and specific about the weight that you wish to be. This is what you will ask for in your mental prompt or mind order. What weight do you want to be?

This is what you will ask for or order for in your mental prompts. You choose your own weight, the weight that you wish to be and then order it by placing it in the unconscious mind where you can retrieve it with your routine motor actions and attitudes in relation to food and eating.

3.4 Exercises For Losing Weight

Here, I present relaxation exercises which will help you to lose weight steadily, easily, effectively, and effortlessly. You do not need to try all of them although you may wish to go through each one of them and settle on the one that makes you feel comfortable. Remember that each of the exercises for losing weight begins with a method for deep relaxation. Follow the procedure which is given above. This procedure is incorporated in the exercises given below.

It is a mental exercise so it is best to start by closing the eyes. This is useful as it enables you to focus on the screen which you will see behind your closed eyelids when you are fully relaxed and in tune with the procedure. Pictures or words may appear on this screen depending on the particular situation and you may also appear on the screen performing a particular exercise. For example, in one of the exercises given below, you are prompted to visualise yourself on the scales or imagine yourself standing in front of a mirror. When you are deeply relaxed and in tune with the situation you will see both the mirror and scale on the screen of your mind.

However, since you are reading the exercises here for the first time, it is quite in order to leave your eyes open so you can see what you are reading. When you have mastered the technique and know exactly what you are doing, you will be able to close your eyes in order to perform the exercises.

Alternatively, you may record the text of the exercises and play them on any media tool so you can close your eyes and listen to your own voice as you play it back. Your mind will absorb it quicker because you are listening to your own voice and the words that I say to you in the texts and the ideas in them become your own thought bricks. For the moment, we can proceed with the exercises as follows.

3.5 Using the Deep Relaxation Technique as a method for Induction

Close your eyes and feel yourself relaxing gently as you keep your eyes firmly closed. Now, imagine or picture, if you can, a scene of peace and tranquillity like waves gushing on a sandy shore, leaves rustling in a gentle breeze or whatever scene represents peace and tranquillity to you.

Remember, that the thoughts, pictures and images you have in your mind most often are the things that will materialise into reality for you as these are charged with energy. Always have the thought of your chosen weight, the weight that you wish to be in mind so that it will materialise into reality for you.

Now, take a long, slow, deep breath through your diaphragm. Hold the breath to a count of five, or ten, or whatever number that is appropriate for you. Now open your mouth gently and breathe out slowly as you relax, relax, relax deeper, and deeper. Feel yourself going deeper, and deeper, and deeper into relaxation, becoming more and more progressively relaxed.

Now, take a second long, slow deep breath through your diaphragm. Hold the breath to a count of five, or ten, or the number that is appropriate for you, as before. Open your mouth gently and breathe out slowly as you let the air out of your body and relax, relax, relax, deeper, and deeper.

Now, take a third long, slow, deep breath through your diaphragm and hold to a count of five, or ten, or any number that is appropriate for you. Now, open your mouth and this time as you let the air out of your body gently, I want you to count the numbers down from eight to zero and relax as you go deeper, and deeper, and deeper, and deeper into relaxation.

3.6 Using the Vibrant Energy of the Sun to Bring Peace and Serenity
Now, that you have completed the breathing exercise, you are ready to learn how to use the vibrant, healing, energy of the light of the sun to relax every part of your body. I will show this to you now. The

advantage of the light of the sun is that it has the following symbolic representations for you.

- ❖ The light of the sun is your cue for instant relaxation so that whenever you bring it over to your body you will be relaxed instantly.
- ❖ The light of the sun brings the sunshine into your life with joy and happiness and makes it a lovely day for you at the moment that you bring it over to your body.
- ❖ The light of the sun is like your light in the dark, it helps you to see your way clearly in wherever you are going or in whatever you are doing and in whatever direction you are going. When you bring it over you will see that the ways to the achievement of your goals are sign posted clearly for you.
- ❖ The light of the sun is a positive light that helps you to achieve positive results in your life.
- ❖ The light of the sun brings peace and serenity to your life.
- ❖ The light of the sun is also a healing light with its vibrant healing energy which heals your mind and body and makes you whole.
- ❖ The light of the sun is a general representation for success in anything you do. It represents good health, happiness, joy, vibrant feeling and liveliness.

Hitherto, I have used the word *'r e l a x'* as your cue for instant relation. Now, I am showing you how to use the light of the sun as your cue for relaxation with its added beneficial representations. The light of the sun is not meant to replace the word *'relax'*. Its introduction gives you a choice. You can use one or the other and, as I have mentioned in chapter one. You can, also, use them together, if you prefer, as in the following example.

Whenever you use the word 'r e l a x', you will be relaxed instantly and as you bring the light of the sun over to your body, you will go deeper, and deeper into a more pleasurable state of relaxation as the healing rays of the light of the sun glow all over your body giving you strength, energy, and vitality so that you will feel absolutely vibrant day by day in every way from now onwards.

Now with all the positive representations of the light of the sun in mind, let us proceed with our relaxation of the mind and body with the power of the light of the sun as follows.

Now, I want you to imagine that you are out in the open air on a beautiful day and you have chosen to be in a park, on a beach, on a holiday. The important thing is to choose a comfortable place to be in your mind, a place which represents for you the very ultimate of peace, joy and total relaxation.

Now, I want you to imagine that the light of the sun is a healing light, a positive light, a light that represents joy, happiness, total fulfilment and every positive thing which you wish to feature in your life. The successful achievement of your goal is represented by the warmth of the healing rays of the light of the sun around you.

The light of the sun symbolises your success, your joy, your happiness and your achievement of the weight that you wish to be. Whenever you bring the light of the sun into your life you feel good instantly because it energises you, it dissolves your worries and your anxieties. The light of the sun is a magical light because it brings success to you instantly, effortlessly. The light of the sun is your cue to instant deep relaxation in mind and body. From this moment onwards, whenever you bring the light of the sun over to your body, you will feel deeply relaxed, instantly.

Now, I want you to remember that you are out in the open air on a beautiful day. Notice, that the light of the sun is warm and shining down through your body and it makes you feel good, positive and relaxed. Stay with that feeling. Notice, that there is clear blue sky and the atmosphere where you are is calm and tranquil with a comforting breeze blowing across your body. You feel peaceful, and deeply relaxed.

Now, I want you to imagine that you can bring the light of the sun to your body. Bring it over now to your right arm and focus it there. Now, feel the healing rays of the light of the sun beaming close to your body like the ray of a torch light and move it from the tips of your fingers all the way up to your shoulders. Move it backwards and forward, up and down until you can feel it in your mind as the warmth of the light of the sun penetrates your skin, your muscles, your nerves and the bones in your body.

As this feeling begins to surge through your body, you can feel your entire body beginning to relax more, and more, deeper, and deeper, becoming more deeply relaxed. The feeling of relaxation will become an everyday feeling for you from this moment onwards. I want you to know that the unconscious mind is acknowledging what is happening now so this feeling of relaxation will become an everyday feeling for you.

Now, move the light of the sun from your right arm to your left arm and from the tips of your fingers to your shoulders. Move it backwards and forward and imagine your left arm going deeply relaxed as your entire body settles down into deep relaxation. As the feeling of relaxation increases in your body and in your life in general, your sense and feeling of peace and tranquillity will also increases accordingly.

Now, I want you to bring the light of the sun over to your right leg and move it from the tips of your toes all the way up to your hip. With each breathe that you take from now onwards, you can feel your muscles relaxing deeply. Your constant deep relaxation will act to dissolve any tensions, worries or anxieties that you may have.

With increased deep relaxation, your mind will be focused on peace and tranquillity from now onwards. This is how things will be for you from now onwards. Notice, that at this moment, the toes of your right leg, your feet, your ankles, lower leg, upper leg and the muscles all the way up to your hip are deeply relaxed, very deeply relaxed.

Now, I want you to turn your attention to your left leg and move the light of the sun from your right leg to your left leg and move it gently from your toes all the way up to your hip and feel your left leg relaxing deeper, and deeper, and deeper.

Now, I want you to notice it as part of your active participation in this exercise, that with both of your legs very, very relaxed and both of your arms very deeply relaxed, you can feel your entire body going deeper, and deeper, and deeper into relaxation with each breath that you take, with each moment you are deeply relaxed, and feeling great. Endeavour to stay with this feeling and make it a daily occurrence for yourself.

I want you to know that, in general, some people feel light and weightless when they are relaxed, as light and weightless as if they can just float away. Other people experience a tingling sensation all over their body while some others have a feeling of elation or a feeling of peace, and contentment.

Whatever feeling you have at this moment should be a positive feeling and this is right and proper for you. Stay with your positive feeling and allow your mind to settle down as you go deeper, deeper, and deeper into relaxation.

Now, I want you to bring the light of the sun over, gently, into your stomach and feel the power of the warm light of the sun inside your body. Feel it now as it glows and energises you. Feel the vibrant energy of the healing light of the sun healing every part of your body as it glows all over you.

You feel positive, confident, and joyful as the healing energy from the light of the sun glows all over your body and this helps you to relax deeper, deeper, and deeper as you become more, and more peaceful. You can feel the peace, and joy which relaxation brings to your life as you notice that the problems and the cares and worries of the day are dissolved by the light of the sun as you go further, and further into deep relaxation.

Now, I want you to turn your attention to your chest and move the light of the sun from your stomach to your chest and feel it glowing over your chest. Notice, that as the light glows over your chest, it penetrates deeper into the internal organs of your body.

Feel it now soothing your heart, feel it moving out into every part of your body and feel every part of your body reacting positively to the power of the healing energy from the light of the sun. You are now feeling very deeply relaxed in mind and body. Notice, that your mind is becoming very peaceful and you have a feeling of joy and happiness. This is how things would be for you from now onwards.

Now, I want you to bring the light of the sun and focus it on the top of your head. I want you to notice that as you do this, your brain channels the healing energy of the light of the sun, once again, to every part of the internal organs in your body. Notice, that when the light gets to your spine, it begins to move out to all areas of your body as it did before.

Feel it now. Feel it as it begins to move to every organ in your body and every organ in your body is becoming active, alive and relaxing deeply. Every organ in your body is becoming healed by the light of the sun and every organ is now working perfectly well as it should. Relax, and allow the healing process to begin in your body, allow the positive changes to take place in your body and in your life from now onwards.

Now, I want you to move the healing light of the sun across your shoulders and feel it relaxing your shoulders and all the muscles around your shoulders and upper arm.

Now, I want you to turn your attention to other parts of your body above your shoulders and notice that your forehead is relaxing deeper, and deeper, your scalp relaxes also and your neck relaxes, the muscles around your eyes relax, your cheeks relax. I want you to allow every part of your face to relax freely and allow yourself to go into a deeper, more joyful, more comfortable state of relaxation.

You are now relaxed, very deeply relaxed. You should feel at ease with what is happening now in your body and very much at ease and contented with the sheer peace and exhilaration that is being made available to you now through this method of deep relaxation. From this moment onwards everything should be as you have planned them because you are making your plans with relaxed peace of mind.

3.7 Using Mental Prompts to Give Instructions to your Mind
In a few moments time you will be giving mental prompts to your unconscious mind asking it to receive certain information or instructions

from you and to act on it as part of your everyday motor actions. These mental prompts will act to strengthen your determination to lose weight, your desire, your will power and your self control. The mental prompts will be invigorating for you in mind and body and will make it possible for you to maintain your natural wholeness and your goal to lose weight.

These mental prompts are the positive instructions which you give to your unconscious mind when you count the numbers down from eight to zero in a few moments. Each and every mental prompt will have a great effect on you in relation to your eating habit and your attitude to food and your health and wellbeing in general. You count down the numbers to go down in body weight as the weights drop off your mind and body just as the weights drop off your mind and body in the prelude exercise at the beginning of this book.

The mental prompts will grow stronger and stronger in you and become more, and more effective for you from this moment onwards as they become imprinted on your unconscious mind. In this way, the mental prompts will become totally a complete part of your everyday motor behaviour, totally and completely effective for you immediately. As they have been imprinted on the unconscious mind, they grow in their strength and effectiveness because each and every time you begin to eat, the unconscious mind will alert you to count the numbers down mentally as the weights drop off your body until you arrive at your correct weight or your chosen weight.

At any time that you do this you find that the mental prompts have a distinctive effect on you. Remember the principle that the ideas which you have most often in your mind will become your reality. Remember the power of the unconscious mind. You may continue the exercise with mental prompts at the moment of ultimate relaxation as follows.

You are now very deeply relaxed, very, very deeply relaxed. Your deep feeling of relaxation ushers in a feeling of peace and contentment which stays with you as the deep relaxation surges through to every part of your body. Now, I want you to imagine that you are back on that beautiful place in the open air where you were a moment ago. I want you to be there at the count of one to three. The count now is one, two, three. You are there.

I want you to notice that the light of the sun is warm and shining down around your body and you have a feeling of peace, tranquillity, and total relaxation. As you continue to relax in this way you will find that through the days and nights from now onwards, with your increased deep relaxation, the weight will begin to drop out of your body and out of your mind steadily, easily, effectively, and effortlessly just as it did in our prelude exercise.

Each and every mental prompt given here will be with you as a constant part of you as part of your motor actions for your mind is being programmed now to receive the mental prompts and you will act on them automatically, involuntarily, unconsciously. You will begin carrying out the dictates of the mental prompts in your motor activities and they will become effective for you immediately. These mental prompts will change your attitude to food and your attitude to eating because you now have much more self control, much more willpower and much more determination to achieve success with your goal of losing weight than ever before.

I want you to stay relaxed and go deeper, deeper, and deeper. I want you to realise from now onwards that with each and every passing day you have the power to obtain whatever you desire. The power to get whatever you desire is truly within you and your desire at this moment is so forceful that you can actually visualize yourself becoming that correct weight that you have chosen for yourself.

Remember your journey to the new world of infinite positive possibilities. You can make that journey again at anytime you choose as it will help you to actualize your goals.

3.8 Further use of the Power of Mental Prompts in Positive Suggestions
Counting the numbers down as the Weights Drop off Your Body, Magically.
You are now very deeply relaxed and ready to give effective mental prompts to your unconscious mind. From this moment onwards, each

and every time you begin to eat your mind will prompt you to take a long, slow deep breath and to count the numbers down from eight to zero.

In counting the numbers down from eight to zero, you imagine yourself bringing the warm light of the sun down around you and relax with the knowledge that from this moment onwards each and every descending number from eight down to zero will be a step down in body weight and each number will have an extra representational meaning for you.

These extra representational meanings are your positive suggestions which act as your mental prompts and they will become more and more effective for you from this moment onwards so that every time you use these mental prompts they will become stronger, and stronger, and stronger, and they will help you to lose weight steadily, easily, effectively, and effortlessly.

Now, I want you to continue to be relaxed as I count down the numbers from eight all the way to zero. As I do this, you will be dropping down, down, down in body weight until you arrive at the correct weight which you have chosen for yourself, the weight that you wish to be. You will be able to maintain your correct weight, the weight that you wish to be, effortlessly. As I count the numbers down, the burden of the extra weight will be lifted off your body and you will become lighter, and lighter, and lighter, in body weight. As you count down from eight to zero, the extra meanings of the numbers will be represented for you in your mental prompts as follows.

*The number now is **eight.** The number eight represents your **effective use of low calorie food and total focus on deep relaxation.***

From this moment onwards, the number eight will become for you, an effective use of low calorie food, and a trigger for deep mental focus on total relaxation. It will remind you to relax totally, completely, mentally, and physically. It stipulates that you eat only because you are truly hungry. The number eight also dictates that you cease from seeking to use food as an oral gratification for other problems in occasions of anxiety.

The number eight eliminates the need to use food as a solution for emotional problems, worries or anxieties. It dissolves your worries, anxieties and it is a detergent to negative thoughts. The number eight makes you an expert in calorie control so that you are a strict calorie controller.

The number eight makes you an efficient and effective user of low calorie food. The use of low calorie food will become a permanent part of your eating habit so you will lose weight steadily, easily, naturally and effectively. You will do so effortlessly because you are doing so in your motor actions, automatically, unconsciously.

As the unconscious mind acknowledges the significance of the number eight to your goal of losing weight, the stipulations and representations of the number eight will become effective for you immediately because they will be acted out in your motor actions in relation to your eating habits.

*The number **seven** represents **losing up to 1,000 calories every day, and the elimination of high calorie food, and junk food.***

As you lose 1,000 calories every day, you will be losing up to 2lb of body weight every week and you will be losing the weight consistently, effortlessly until you reach your correct weight, the weight which you have chosen to be. I want you to feel yourself going deeper, deeper, and deeper into relaxation, moving down, down, down in body weight and as this happens you can feel the extra weight beginning to drop off slowly from your body until you lose them all consistently, steadily, and completely.

From now onwards losing weight becomes a big gain in your self confidence so as you become more, and more confident you will lose the weight steadily and at a rate which is consistent with the health and natural wholeness of your body.

As every mental prompt is recorded in your unconscious mind, the elimination of junk food and high calorie food from your life will take place automatically in your motor actions in relation to your attitudes towards food from now onwards. From this moment onwards, junk food and high calorie food will be out of your life for good.

Your perception of high calorie food and junk food will change from now onwards as they begin to appear terrifyingly loathsome and repulsive to you. From the moment of the unpleasantness of these foods, they will cease to feature in your consciousness. As these food begin to look repulsive and unpleasant to you, they will be eliminated completely from your eating habits.

The number seven means that high calorie food and junk food will be eliminated totally from your consciousness. Instead of those foods, you will now begin to enjoy a greater variety of food. You will eat more fruits and vegetables, more wholesome and natural food. You will be happy and eager to eliminate high calorie food and junk food from your life because you are a health conscious person.

You know that when you eliminate high calorie food and junk food you will be reducing the risk of the health problems associated with those foods. You will know that with the elimination of those kinds of food, your health will improve day by day in every way.

*The number **six** represents your **losing weight, looking good and feeling great.***

I want you to notice that with the number six in this counting down exercise, as each pound of weight leaves your body you will find that you have more energy, more vitality, more joy of living and of life. You are relaxed now, very much more relaxed and at peace with yourself.

From this moment onwards, you will sustain the need to look good and feel great while losing weight by a consistent course of light exercises such as the mental exercises in this book because you know that the more and more you exercise your mind and body, the more alert, fitter, stronger and healthier you become. In this way, you will gain more strength, energy and stamina which are necessary requirements in your regime of losing weight.

Now, relax and focus your mind on your objectives in relation to losing weight. Allow your mind to drift deeper, deeper, and become more, and more relaxed. Each and every time you use these mental prompts you will find that they have become a permanent, total part of you because they have been imprinted on your unconscious mind.

*The number **five** represents that **you are eating less and less food and enjoying it more and more as you feel easily full up with smaller amount of food than before.***

Allow your mind to relax now and go deeper, deeper, and deeper, easily, effortlessly into relaxation. I want you to know this to your benefit that because your unconscious mind retains all the information which it receives, the positive mental prompts which it receives about losing weight will help you to lose weight steadily, easily, effectively, and effortlessly. You will be able to maintain your correct weight, the weight that you have chosen to be, and a healthy body.

The positive mental prompts are the systems programme for your unconscious mind to help you so that from now onwards you will eat only the food that is necessary to make you feel good and look great, the food that is necessary for the health and natural wholeness of your body. Everything else that is unnecessary for your health will be unpleasant and repulsive in its taste and appearance to you so it will be eliminated for everything that you eat from now onwards will only be the food that is necessary to make your body feel healthy and look beautiful.

As you are deeply relaxed now, I want you to look closely on the screen of your mind. Notice the picture of how you want to be, notice that you have a shapely and attractive body, a well proportioned body. This is pleasing to you so you will maintain your body and keep it healthy and attractive always by eating low calorie healthy food.

From this moment onwards, you will start on a systematic health conscious regime of detoxification to rid your body of the effects of high calorie food. As the high calorie food is eliminated from your life, you will be able to lose 1,000 calories day by day as you are eating less and less junk food and high calorie food and you will be looking great, feeling good and happier and happier day by day in every way.

*The number **four** represents that **you are losing your appetite for food and your hunger is quenched easily as you are eating less and less but you are feeling good and looking great at all times.***

From this moment onwards you will eat your food without rushing yourself. You will take time to eat your food and to enjoy it and digest it well. As you are losing 1,000 calories day by day, you are eating only what is necessary for your health. Therefore, you will be losing weight more and more, steadily, easily, effectively and effortlessly.

As you are only eating low calorie healthy food, you are feeling good and looking great as you lose weight. You love yourself for the way you look and feel for losing weight means gaining a strong, healthy and attractive body and attaining the weight that you have set for yourself, the weight that you wish to be.

As you continue to lose weight, you will be ,feeling good and looking great and you will be happy with the success that you are achieving with your goal and happy with the way that you are making necessary changes to your life. The glowing force of the healing light of the sun will energise you and give you the strength and vitality to resist any temptation to indulge in an unwanted eating.

Now, I want you to relax and imagine that you are drifting deeper, deeper becoming more and more progressively relaxed. From this moment onwards you will begin to feel extremely light and weightless and very, very pleased with your achievement in losing weight steadily, easily, effectively and effortlessly. In this way, you will look good and feel great.

*Number **three** represents that **you are leaving food constantly on your plate at meal times because you are satisfied with smaller portions.***

As you are losing your appetite for food and your hunger is quenched easily, quickly, you leave food unfinished on your plate on a regular and consistent basis. You leave food unfinished on your plate when you eat at home, when you eat in hotels on holidays, when you eat in restaurants and at parties. You leave food unfinished on your plate everyday whatever food you eat. Your unconscious mind recognises your actions and imprints it as a motor activity for you so that you can lose weight easily and effortlessly. You feel good about your actions and you look great in your appearance.

As you are feeling good and looking great, you derive immense pleasure and satisfaction from leaving unfinished meal on your plate because this indicates that you are full up by eating less and less day by day in every way. This also indicates the power of your unconscious mind in making the routine of leaving unfinished food on your plate a motor action for you.

The success which you are achieving from this action increases your will power, your determination to succeed and you self control in resisting any temptation for indulgence with food. Now, I want you to relax, go deeper, deeper and deeper into a feeling of total relaxation.

*Number **two** represents that **you are able to visualise yourself now as you would look when all the excess weight is cast off your body.***

I want you to relax, go deeper, deeper and deeper into total relaxation. I want you to look again at the screen on your mind and, this time, look at it closely and see yourself on the screen, looking as you would like to be. I want you to notice that you look great on the screen, you look pretty or handsome and attractive and you feel good watching that screen.

This picture is in your mind and you have the power right now to make it your reality because the picture and thoughts which you have in your mind most often will become your reality through the power of your unconscious mind and your motor actions.

I want you to feel the radiant energy of the healing light from the sun moving through your body and energising you. Feel it now and remember that the light from the sun is a positive light, a healing light, a magical light which enables you to accomplish whatever you wish to accomplish. Feel the light now descending to the top of your head, moving down into your body, moving through your spine, moving out from your spine into every organ in your body, moving into every part of your body.

You now feel completely relaxed. The light from the sun heals your body and makes you whole. Now, every part of your body radiates the peace, joy, happiness, love and harmony from the light of the sun. I want you to remember our fundamental principle that there is no limit to what you can achieve with the power of your mind except the restrictions which you impose on yourself by negative acts of self doubt.

Your unconscious mind will always guide and protect you against the temptation of negative thoughts and self doubt. It will also, help you to avoid the temptation of eating junk food, unhealthy food and unnecessary food in general from this moment onwards.

*Number **one** represents that **you know now that all the mental prompts have been recorded in your unconscious mind and will become part of your motor actions and they will be completely effective for you from this moment onwards.***

From this moment onwards you will be losing weight gradually, consistently day by day in every way. Always remember that your body is obedient to your mind. All the mental prompts have been acknowledged by your conscious and unconscious mind and as a result of this the mental prompts will surface in your motor actions. You will lose weight steadily, easily and effectively and you will do so effortlessly. In this way you will look good and feel great, always.

You will begin today to cut down on your calorie intake and you will be losing 1,000 calories day by day in every way. As you lose these calories you will be able to lose up to 2lb of body weight every week. As a result of this, the positive changes that you require in your appearance will come steadily, easily, consistently and effectively and these positive changes will be noticed by your family, friends, the people you work with or the people around you in general. You will look good and feel great.

*The count **zero** it is accomplished. The count zero represents **the accomplishment of your goal. It means that the goal of losing weight has now been accomplished, that you are now losing weight steadily, easily, and effectively and that you are doing so effortlessly because the mental prompts have all been imprinted on your unconscious mind and you are always relaxed in mind and body.***

You have now acquired a relaxed attitude in mind and body in anything you do from day to day from this moment onwards. You are now relaxed, very, very deeply relaxed. You are happy with the knowledge that you made a goal to lose weight and you derive an immense benefit from your goal as you are now losing weight. As you continue to achieve success with your goal of losing weight, you will be happy with your knowledge and mastery of our mind technique and much happier that you have lost weight steadily, easily, effectively, and you have done so effortlessly. In doing so, you will be feeling good and looking great.

Now as you continue to relax day by day in every way and focus your mind on your objective of losing weight, you will find that with your increased relaxation, the weight has begun to drop off consistently out of your body and out of your mind until you attain the weight that you have chosen for yourself, the weight that you wish to be. As you are in a relaxed mood and in control of your life day by day from this moment onwards, you will be able to maintain your chosen weight, that weight that you wish to be.

Through the days and through the nights from now onwards your mind will be focused on peace and contentment in the knowledge that everything is working well for you in accordance with your action plans for losing weight. As the burden of the unwanted extra weight drops off your body, you are free from the pressure of carrying the extra weight and you now feel very light and weightless, as light and weightless as if you can float away. This is a very pleasant feeling for you and it is the way things would be for you from this moment onwards.

Now, I want you to bring the healing light of the sun around you as a weapon to guard you and protect you against the temptation to overindulge in food from now onwards. Bring it over gently to the top of your head. Allow it to relax you and release you from negative thoughts. Allow it to cleanse your mind and body generally and make you more and more confident in your ability to lose weight.

Through the days and through the nights from this moment onwards you will have much more energy and vitality as the result of your positive decision and effort to effect changes in your life. You will be happier by it knowing that with the loss of the burden of excess weight, you will look prettier or handsome, healthier and much more attractive than ever before.

I am now going to count the numbers to you upwards from one to five. With each and every ascending number the energy from the healing light of the sun will increase within your body and you will open your eyes (if they are closed now as advised at the beginning of the exercise) at the count of five.

You will be feeling very alert, refreshed and really feeling on top of the world. You will be able to face the rest of the day (or night) with renewed happiness, joy, strength, energy and vitality in the knowledge that your goal has been accomplished. You will be able to feel this way from day to day from this moment onwards.

1. I want you to feel the healing energy of the light of the sun surging through your body. Feel it now as it moves into every part of your body as you are slowly getting ready to come out of the state of deep relaxation.

2. I want you to begin now to move your hands and feet slowly as you come out from the state of deep relaxation. You are feeling very alert to your immediate environment, feeling alive and happy as a little smile begins to form on your face. This indicates a feeling of wellbeing.

3. You are now making some movements in your body, feeling good, coming out of the state of deep relaxation with the knowledge that you are now losing weight easily, steadily, effectively and effortlessly. You will look good and feel great regularly from now onwards.

4. You now have a broad smile on your face, a great feeling of wellbeing and a clear picture of the new you with the correct weight which you have chosen for yourself. The weight that you wish to be will become your real weight as you continue to feel light and weightless from day to day.

5. The number now is five. You can open your eyes now and sit up with a clear knowledge that you are beginning to lose weight now and will continue to do so steadily, easily, effectively, and effortlessly until you reach your correct weight, the weight that you have chosen for yourself, the weight that you wish to be. This will become your real weight and you will be able to maintain this weight, feel good and look great from now onwards.

3.9 How to Make Your Dream Weight Your Reality

You can lose weight steadily, easily, and effectively by making your dream weight a reality. Remember that the thoughts which you have most often in your mind will become your reality. If you can bring your thoughts into pictures and see them clearly then you can realise them easily and effortlessly. This is one way in which your dreams become your reality.

I mentioned earlier on in this chapter that you will be prompted later to visualize yourself on the scales or imagine yourself standing in front of a mirror. I will now show you how to do this exercise here. In this relaxation exercise, you will learn how to picture your desires and realise them. Remember also the journey to the world of infinite positive possibilities in the preparatory exercise in chapter one. You can make the journey any time you wish as it will help you to achieve your goals and any other aspirations that you might have.

3.10 Relaxation Exercise

Follow the steps as in the previous section.

Now, I want you to have a clear image, in your mind, of yourself standing on the scales and the scales registering the correct weight that you have chosen for yourself, the weight that you wish to be. Alternatively you may wish to have a clear image of yourself fitting into the size of clothing that you wish to fit into.

See this image very clearly for this is the weight that you have chosen for yourself, the weight that you wish to be, this is the weight that you will be. See yourself looking the way that you would like to look with the extra weight taken off those parts of your body where you want the weight to be taken off.

Remember the first principle that the thoughts which you have most often in your mind will become your reality. To make this possible for you in relation to losing weight, I want you now to visualize yourself looking at yourself in the mirror and seeing the image of yourself as you would like to be. See this image very, very vividly and summon this image into your mind many times during the day particularly just after waking up in the morning, before eating any meal, and before going to bed at night. Remember always, that this is the way you wish to look, this is the weight that you wish to be. Believe it strongly and let this image of yourself stay in the unconscious mind so that it will become your reality.

Remember always, my discussions of the fundamental principles of mind power. When you have attained the weight that you have chosen for yourself, the weight that you wish to be which is represented by the image which you see on the screen of your mind at this moment, you will be able to maintain it, you will find yourself eating just enough to maintain your desired weight.

Until you attain this weight, you will find that you have less and less desire to eat between meals. From now onwards, you will be content with eating smaller meals than before, so you will be eating less and less but feeling good, looking great and healthy because you are eating only healthy food.

As you begin to derive great satisfaction from eating smaller but healthy, low calorie, meals you will find that your desire for high calorie unhealthy food has been eliminated from your life. As you lose weight and approach closer and closer to the weight that you have chosen for yourself, the weight that you wish to be, you will find yourself growing stronger and stronger, healthier and healthier day by day in every way. Your resistance to illness and disease will increase day by day because you are eating for the health and natural wholeness of your body.

With the loss of the burden of excess weight you will feel better and better and your health will become better and better. From this moment onwards, as you lose weight and your health continues to improve, you will be more motivated to do some regular simple exercises such as the relaxation exercises which are given here in this book. This will also make you feel better and better because the more and more you relax and use your mind and body the stronger and stronger they become and your health will improve generally in every way.

Every so often, you will replace eating a meal with some type of exercise. You have set a goal for yourself with regard to attaining the weight that you have chosen for yourself, the weight that you wish to be. You will find that you are able to regulate and monitor your eating habit and your calorie control so that you lose weight accordingly and achieve and maintain the weight that you have chosen for yourself, the weight that you wish to be.

You will remember your deliberations on the effects of being overweight. This deliberation revealed to you some of the serious health and social issues involved in being overweight. The knowledge from your deliberation made your journey to the world of positive possibilities a necessary journey. You will be more and more aware of the undesirable effect of being overweight and you will take effective action in the knowledge that action is the route to change and progress in the goal of losing weight.

When a health conscious person is heavier than expected, the excess weight brings with it a deep feeling of embarrassment for the person as the person is made uncomfortable because of the excess weight. The person's appearance suffers and the health of the person is threatened. However, as a health conscious person, the individual knows that the embarrassment and the uncomfortable feeling are a great spur for positive action to change the existing situation.

With this in mind, you will act with positive action in the knowledge that action is the route to change. With positive action you will derive pleasure in the knowledge that achieving and maintaining the weight that you have chosen for yourself, the weight that you wish to be, will be accomplished to your satisfaction and fully accomplished effortlessly because your positive thinking and positive actions in relation to your goal of losing weight have been recognised by your unconscious mind.

You will be losing your appetite for eating between meals and other unnecessary eating habits that you might have. As a result of this, you will be eating only at your regular meal times when you are hungry. From now onwards you will be eating less and less food because your hunger is satisfied quickly by eating smaller meals.

You leave unfinished food on your plate regularly because you are eating less and less yet you are in good health because you are eating low calorie healthy food. Therefore, you will feel good and look great. Your unconscious mind will help you to maintain the weight that you have chosen for yourself, the weight that you wish to be and this will help you to continue to feel good and look great day by day in every way.

I want you to know that your body is always obedient to the dictates of your mind. Your unconscious mind is now programmed with the mental prompts given here and it will help you to change your eating habits in order to make your weight loss easier for you. It will eliminate any junk food and high calorie food from your consciousness and from your eating habit. In this way, it will help you to eat for the health and the natural wholeness of your body. You will be eating low calorie healthy foods, you will be healthy and you will continue to feel good and look great, always.

As you continue to eat low calorie healthy food, you will notice that you are becoming calm with each and every passing day, more confident day by day in every way. Your increasing calmness, confidence, determination and self control will help you to eliminate the temptation for unnecessary eating.

As you continue to relax day by day in every way, you will find that, as before, you have less and less appetite for food and your hunger is satisfied quickly and easily by eating smaller meals, fruits, vegetables, day by day from now onwards. In this way, you will be able to achieve and maintain your desired weight easily and effortlessly.

Now, as I count the numbers upwards from 1 to 5, you will sit up at the count of 5 and you will feel very lively, full of strength, energy, and vitality and the feelings will stay with you and be part of your everyday feeling from this moment onwards. At the count of 5, you will feel it and know it that you are losing weight steadily, easily and effortlessly. When you arrive at the weight that you have chosen for yourself, the weight that you wish to be, you will be able to maintain it for as long as you want. The count now is number one, two, three, four, five.

3.11 Going for Your Success in Losing Weight with Confidence

If you have followed, attentively, everything that I have discussed with you here so far, then you have grasped the essential ingredients in the recipe for success in the use of your mind to get what you want. Always remember that whatever success you achieve in whatever field comes through your effective use of your mind in the sense that thinking precedes and provokes action.

You must now consolidate on what you have gained from this book. To do this you must display confidence in yourself and in your ability to succeed in your chosen field, that is, in your ability to lose weight steadily, easily, effectively and to do so effortlessly with the power of the unconscious mind.

You can display your new found confidence by translating the secrets you have found in this book, your new found pattern of belief system, your new wealth of ideas, your positive attitudes and positive frame of mind in respect to yourself and your goals and aspiration, and so on, into action. Do not be afraid to seek to achieve success, be resolute in your desire to achieve success in losing weight.

I have discussed various mind techniques for losing weight in this chapter and various methods of relaxation in this book right from the beginning with the preparatory exercise which set the psychical system in motion for you. Use the method that suits you and practise the exercise that you feel most comfortable with but you must practise because action is the route to change.

Action is the essential ingredient that brings success in any goal and constant practise makes one perfect in any exercise for personal improvement. Now, you must take the bull by the horn with courage and boldness and you will be successful in your goal. Do not procrastinate for this is negative thinking. I say to you, **go for it with confidence so that you can Lose Weight Now!**

Believe me, you can be a great success in any venture if you think you can. You must think constructive thoughts supported by positive action. I mentioned the *Cogito* of Rene Descartes in the first chapter of this book to illustrate the power of thought. Now here is a new slant to the Cogito.

I think that I have the power within me, the power of belief, to lose weight steadily, easily, effectively, and effortlessly, therefore, I can lose weight now!

Now think about the force of that statement and the spirit of determination in it, articulate it by action, doing something new. Remember the principles of mind power, if you truly believe that you can do it then, so be it, you can. Remember that a true belief in the sense of 'belief' in this book, is one that is like faith and ignites serious positive action.

3.12 Practice Sessions
How to Give Yourself a Confidence Booster
Follow the method which I have discussed above and proceed with personal instructions about what is to be done, then follow up with

deep relaxation and finally, the essential positive mental prompts at the moment of ultimate relaxation.

As I have already suggested, above, in this chapter, if you think it is more convenient, you may record the texts of the exercises on any media tool which you can playback and listen to regularly. Your mind will absorb the messages quicker because in listening to the messages you will be listening to your own voice, the ideas become your own thought bricks and the effect of listening to them is astonishingly therapeutic.

I give you a further guide here with more exercises. As before, the procedure is the same order but different words, different pictorial representations and different imagery so you have many to choose from each of the chapters of this book. You may proceed as follows.

Instructions

To begin with, find yourself a very comfortable position, sitting or lying down and proceed as follows. Put yourself into a state of deep relaxation in accordance with the methods which I have demonstrated in this book. While remaining in this relaxed state, give yourself positive mental prompts for the idea of success in losing weight. You may proceed as follows.

Relaxation

Take a long, slow, deep breath through your diaphragm and hold it to a mental count of five. Now open your mouth slowly and gently exhale all the air from your body as you allow the feeling of relaxation to spread through your body from the top of your head all the way down to the tips of your toes. As you relax, you will think positive thoughts about success in losing weight steadily, easily, effectively, and effortlessly. Now, go deeper, deeper, and deeper into peace, going into a higher state of consciousness in relation to the idea of losing weight, feeling good, and looking great.

You may use the vibrant energy of the healing light of the sun to relax every part of your body by mentally bringing it over to any part of your body and commanding it to relax that part of your body as I showed you in exercises above in section 3.6. Alternatively, you may use the exercise where I showed you how to instruct your unconscious mind to accept the word *r e l a x* as your instant cue to relaxation. Now when you have reached the stage of ultimate relaxation and you feel all loosened up, then you proceed to your mental prompts as follows.

Positive Mental Prompts

From this moment onwards, you will think positive thoughts so that positive feelings will flow to you in relation to your success in losing weight steadily, easily, and effectively. You have let go your tense hold on negative thoughts, and negative emotions and you have let go past disappointments, if any, in your life. The past will cease to bother you from now onwards because you have great confidence in yourself and in your plans for losing weight now!

You have planned the way you want to live your life, you have chosen a correct weight for yourself, the weight that you wish to be and the future will be exactly what you want it to be, it will be according to your plans. You will lose weight steadily, easily, and effectively, you will look good, and feel great from now onwards.

You have eliminated restrictive mental frameworks relating to the idea of success in losing weight steadily, easily, and effectively. You have let go mistaken beliefs relating to what you want to achieve so your success in losing weight will come to you through your positive thoughts and attitudes.

Your mind is now clearly attuned to success in your chosen goal so your goal to lose weight will be achieved steadily, easily, and effectively. You are genuinely and seriously concerned with success. You will achieve success because you are a determined person. You are firm and resolute in your search for success so you will derive a great satisfaction from accomplishing your goal of losing weight.

Day by day in every way from now onwards, as you relax you will find that the road to success in your goal of losing weight is clearly sign posted for you, and you will get there and walk on the road of success and arrive happily at your destination which is the accomplishment of your goal of losing weight. You know that success in losing weight steadily, easily, and effectively is possible for you because everything is possible with the power of your mind.

From this moment onwards, everyday in every way as you relax more and more, you will find that relaxation will give you the peace of mind and the inner tranquillity which will enable you to develop much more confidence in yourself and also much more confidence in your ability to do the things that matter in your life, the things that will bring greater success to you in losing weight steadily, easily, and effectively.

From this moment onwards you will be self-reliant. You are now full of independence and a determination to achieve success in your goal to lose weight. You have a great inner courage to succeed. Feel it now. Listen to your inner self. Everyday in every way from this moment onwards you will become more and more self confident as each day brings success to you in whatever you do from day to day.

You will begin now to project a new, positive, self image and you will be successful. As success begins to take over in your life, you will find that you will be much more happy and contented with what you are doing, much more cheerful and much more optimistic about your future in relation to your goal to lose weight. You will use your mind much more clearly and effectively as you come to appreciate the enormous power of your mind to bring success into your life. You will know it to be true that the magic of success is truly within you.

You have mastered the fundamental principles of the mind technique in this book and the secrets of how the human mind works. You have mastered the formulation of goals and the plans of action which will bring the goal about as we have discussed here. You have mastered our techniques of deep relaxation and the effective use of mental prompts and you are adept with the use of breathing exercises to bring calmness and serenity in moments of tension.

As a result of all these great knowledge that you possess, you can now make decisions easily, readily, and correctly in relation to your goals or any aspirations you might have. As the decisions which you make bring successes into your life with each and every passing day, you will find that your life is filled with rich and excitingly rewarding things to do to bring you further success, joy and happiness. So, go for it now with confidence and you will be for ever successful in losing weight steadily, easily, effectively, and effortlessly.

3.13 Affirmations to Bring the Results that You Desire

Affirmations to Maintain Your Chosen Weight

Affirmations have truly magical powers which bring desired results to genuine seekers of success. I have been stating the general rule with affirmations all through this book.

The rule is that you must always affirm what you want to achieve, not the negation of what you want to achieve. You must not affirm the things, conditions or state of affairs which you do not require in your life. Remember the problems of the *Chocolate Cake Lady* in chapter two above.

In brief you must always affirm your wishes, desires, intentions, goals, and so on, and not the negation of your desire or intention. You must never deal with the negation of your intentions for this is negative thinking. It is negative because it is a negation. Remember that the rule is to affirm, at all times, what you really want.

There is a popular statement that people make with good intentions, generally. This Statement is that, "Nothing is Impossible". This serves as affirmation for those making them. However, following our rules for affirmations here in respect of the working of the unconscious mind, the popular statement is a negative affirmation. It is dealing with "Nothing," and "Impossible".

If there is a genuine intention in your affirmation, you will want your affirmations to relate to something which has a possibility of fulfilment. This is the reason why you are making the affirmation.

However, you will notice that "Nothing," and "Impossible" are not the terms which are appropriate for the description of what you wish to achieve or accomplish. Under such circumstances the appropriate affirmation should be that, *"Everything is Possible"*.

Here you are dealing with possibilities. Any goal, wish, or desire that an individual might wish to accomplish is something which is within the realm of possibility and it is entailed by "everything".

With the above rule in mind, try to examine the following statements in respect of the intentions of the individual.

(A) *I am not unhappy, I do not want to be unhappy and I am not tense and not nervous.*
(B) *I am a confident, positive, and optimistic person who is happy, cheerful and relaxed at all times.*

Notice, that (A) is a negative affirmation which should be avoided at all times because this is the affirmation of the negative traits which you must always guard against. On the other hand, (B) is a positive affirmation of the qualities and moods which you wish to retain in your life. You must always avoid the temptation to make affirmations in the form of (A).

Affirmations are very powerful thought bricks of the mind. They work because they follow the principles of mind power which I discussed in the first chapter of this book. They are part of the thought bricks which form the structures of the mind castle which you wish to build. This means that what you affirm is what you get. The statement that forms your affirmation is your declaration, something which you have endorsed or ratified.

Affirmation of Action
This has to do with a planned positive action which will result in the achievement of a desired goal. An individual may have difficulty in obtaining a job or in losing weight. In such situations, such as the present purpose of losing weight, the appropriate affirmations which the individual should make would be made as follows.

I will perform simple physical exercises everyday in order to be fit and healthy.
I will always make determined and resolute plans from now onwards.
I will always finish whatever I start because I start with constructive plans of action.

Whenever I make a plan to do something, I see it to the end.
From this moment onwards I will always eat low calorie healthy food.
I am positive and confident that I will lose weight steadily, easily, and effectively.
I will lose weight now!

In these affirmations you are affirming your determination to lose weight, affirming the result of your determination, that is, that you will lose weight now! What happens is that when you have made the affirmation with real commitment and genuine feelings, as opposed to when you merely verbalise them, unfeelingly, and disinterestedly, parrot fashion, the positive nature of the affirmation will stir your mind to positive action which is expressed in your continued positive thoughts and positive attitudes towards your goal to lose weight.

You can use affirmation of action for whatever goal you wish to accomplish. You make a firm resolve as appropriate to your goal and affirm accordingly, in a determined way. For example, the *Chocolate Cake Lady* could affirm the details in the action plans which I drew up for her in chapter two.

With respect to losing weight, the result of the combined mental operations is that you will be losing weight steadily, easily, effectively, and you will be doing so effortlessly because your unconscious mind acknowledges your good intentions. Remember also the principles of mind power, if you think it and believe it, you will get it because the thought and the belief will provoke you to effective positive action.

Affirmation of Thought Bricks
This is mental affirmation. In this affirmation, you use thought bricks with which to construct your mind castles. You make such affirmations mentally to yourself. For example as I have just mentioned above regarding my illustration in chapter two, *The Chocolate Cake Lady*

may affirm the statements of plans 1 and 2 and repeat it constantly to herself and then back up the mental affirmation with positive action to improve her physical appearance. On the other hand, an individual may affirm the idea of success in general and the result of success as follows.

I am a successful man (woman).
I am always in control of my life.
I know what I want and how to get it.
I will get what I am looking for because what I am looking for is available to me.
I will attain the weight that I want to be because I have chosen the weight for myself.
I will lose weight steadily, easily, and effectively from now until I attain the weight which I have chosen for myself, the weight that I wish to be.

If this affirmation is made constantly it will be retained in the unconscious mind and this will open up new ways for achieving success in the individual's life and ways of accomplishing the goal to lose weight steadily, easily, effectively and effortlessly.

Written Affirmations
This can take the form of a written out positive plan of what the individual wishes to accomplish in his or her life. Remember that I mentioned in the last chapter that a goal that is well formulated must be kept constantly in mind. The best way to do this is to affirm the goal constantly. This makes the goal easily amenable to fulfilment.

Take care and affirm confidently and you will be successful in your goal. Remember the five principles which I discussed in chapter one together with the secrets of how the human mind works. Endeavour to apply your knowledge of those principles and the workings of the mind in everything you do from day to day. I expect that from this moment onwards, you will be looking good and feeling great, always.

CHAPTER FOUR: RECAPITULATION OF SOME ESSENTIAL POINTS

As a follow up to my discussions on affirmations and a fitting conclusion to this book, I wish to recapitulate with you, some of the essential points which I have discussed in this book. These will help you to remember the fun exercises, and also help you to remember the essential points which are necessary for building your confidence. They will make you more determined to lose weight now!

4.1 The Logic of Numbers

Always remember that the logic of numbers determines your success in whatever you do. The more times you practise all the exercises in this book the better chance you will have of achieving your objective of losing weight. Remember the saying, *practise makes perfect*. You will become perfect in whatever you do the more times you practise on it. Let us illustrate with practical affairs as follows.

Suppose that you are an athlete and you want to improve your personal best (PB) performance on your event. The logic of numbers stipulates that the more times your practise, the more proficient you will become in your event. On the other hand, let us suppose that you are looking for a job. The logic of numbers stipulates that if you send out 100 job applications every week your chance of being invited for an interview would be much better than if you send out one job application every week

Remember the saying, *If, at first, you don't succeed, try, try and try again.* This saying implicates the logic of numbers as it is a statement of determined achievers. Perseverance, like persistence, is part of the logic of numbers because it shows an individual's determination to succeed in a chosen objective.

You may also have heard of the famous French Emperor, Napoleon Bonaparte 1 (1769-1821) who fought and won many battles until his defeat by the British soldier and statesman, Arthur Wellesley (1769-1852)

the first Duke of Wellington, at the battle of Waterloo in 1815. Napoleon was reputedly attributed with the statement that "Victory belongs to the most persevering." I rest my case.

The principle of the logic of numbers is a doctrine for determined achievers. The principle is easy to understand and simple to apply in our daily routines. The principle of the logic of numbers is implicated in a general way in the fundamental principles of thought bricks which I discussed in the first part of this book.

When you have positive thoughts about your objective of losing weight and practise the mental exercises in this book, you will find that you will lose weight steadily, easily, and effectively. You will do so effortlessly when your goal to lose weight has been imprinted on your unconscious mind.

4.2 The Magic of Success

Always remember that the thought bricks for success in any venture are constructed in the mind. In any situation, if you think you can, you are already on your way to the winning post. It is all in the state of the mind. Your success in anything you do begins in your mind. This is the essence of mind power. The mind is the magic power that a person can use to achieve great success in whatever he or she does. Thus, you must always attune your mind to success and you will be successful in whatever you do. Remember that *the magic of success is truly within you.* It is within your mind. Apply the magic now in your attempt to lose weight and you will notice that the weight will drop off your body, magically.

4.3 The Pitfalls of Negative Prompts

Always think positive thoughts about your goals. When you give mental prompts to yourself or whenever you make affirmations about your goal of losing weight, use positive words that enhance your desire. As I have mentioned in my discussions of affirmations above, you must always affirm your objectives or whatever you wish to achieve and avoid the temptation to use negative expressions in talking about your goal. Examine the following illustrations.

(A) *During tomorrow's meeting I will not be tired and I will not be sleepy.*
(B) *I will not fail to lose weight.*

You will notice that (A) and (B) above are very negative expressions in terms of what you wish to accomplish. The illustration (A) is about tiredness and sleepiness and (B) is talking about failure. In consideration of what you want to achieve the correct, positive, affirmation should be as follows.

(C) During tomorrow's meeting I will be wide awake, alert and energetic.
(D) I will lose weight steadily, easily, effectively, and effortlessly.

Notice that (C) and (D) above show more determination than (A) and (B). When your instructions, affirmations, or mental prompts are made in an emphatic way as (C) and (D) they become more effective for you.

If you wish to know more about the practical effects of negative prompts refer to my previous book (Maurice-Nneke 2002, pages 174-176)

4.4 Action is the Route to Change

As I stated in the introductory chapter, any person who is able to talk the talk about a goal of losing weight must be prepared to walk the walk to realize the goal by putting the talk into positive action. Action is necessary to bring about the changes that you require. If you fail to act then no changes will be made to the existing situation and the lack of change will be due to your lack of action.

If you have a genuine, serious, intention of losing weight then you owe it to yourself to perform all the necessary actions as advised in this book. Remember the principles of the action plan which I drew out for the *Chocolate Cake Lady* in chapter two above and draw out a similar action plan to suit your purpose.

Remember, that a positive action is a positive expression of thought, and always avoid the temptation to finger point and blame others such as the supermarkets or the food manufacturers for the high calorie food that you have been eating. Remember, that low calorie food is there as a choice for you and take the responsibility to change your eating habit because it matters to you. Always endeavour to do something to effect a change in the particular situation which you are concerned with. You can refer now to my discussion of the fundamental principles of the mind power technique in chapter one in my discussion of the topic, *'Action is the Route to Change'*.

4.5 Belief is the Ultimate

Belief is an essential ingredient in a recipe for success in anything you do. You can be a great success in any venture if you believe that you can. Remember, that no one is ready for success in any goal or venture until he or she believes that he or she can be successful in the particular goal or venture.

Remember, also, that belief is the opposite of doubt. When you have belief you always pursue your goal with a determination to attain the goal. Your belief is a thought brick. You must think constructive thoughts supported by positive actions that affirm your belief. For the purpose of losing weight, which is the subject of this book, a statement of belief can be expressed as follows.

- ❖ I will lose weight steadily, easily, and effortlessly and attain the weight that I have chosen for myself, the weight that I wish to be; because success is guaranteed to me by my belief that I will attain the weight that I wish to be.
- ❖ I can get whatever I am looking for because I believe that I can.
- ❖ I will lose weight steadily, easily, effectively, and effortlessly because I believe that I can.

When you are able to make such statements as the above in relation to your goals and aspirations, you will know for certain that you are on the way to achieving your objective. I am concerned here with genuine belief so the above statements are not meant to be mere verbal utterances. Notice, that in the above statements, the action words, that is the words constituting the actions, such as *attain, get, lose* are all affirmed by the belief.

For the particular purpose of losing weight it is important that you have your belief as a mental theory of success. This ensures that when you genuinely believe that you can lose weight now, your belief guarantees your success in losing weight because your belief has been retained in the unconscious mind as a positive and highly effective thought brick. This means that, for you, success in losing weight exists as a thought process in your mind and that you are aware of this.

You can see clearly from what I have stated variously here, that when such thought process has taken hold in the unconscious mind, the individual's attitude towards success in losing weight, or in any particular venture, betrays the existence of positive thoughts about losing weight and about success in general. Such individual is often confident, positive and optimistic in personal situations and circumstances.

When you experience such a situation you know that you are on your way to success because your positive attitude towards your goal clearly manifests your confidence and your success is guaranteed by your belief which induces your positive action. You can refer now to my discussion of belief in chapter one to help you to have a rock solid belief in yourself and in your ability to achieve success in your goal of losing weight.

In this way the thought brick which entails your goal is always with you, always in your mind. As you know from my discussions about goals, in order to achieve success with the goal of losing weight, the goal must be kept constantly in your mind at all times otherwise you may run the risk of supplanting it with some other wish or desire. Thus, as a final checkpoint, you must practise the following exercises to help you with your goal of losing weight and any other goal or venture which you may have.

4.6 Key Points to Remember
- ❖ Practise the preparatory exercise in chapter one and try to make the journey to the world of positive possibilities as often as you wish for the achievement of any goal or venture that you might have.

- ❖ Practise the relaxation exercises in this book and master the procedure as presented from the breathing exercise, the relaxation of your mind and body and the essential mental prompts that will help you to achieve your objectives.
- ❖ Learn the five fundamental principles of our mind power technique and the secrets of how the human mind works and apply them appropriately in what you do from day to day.
- ❖ Refer to my discussion of goals in chapter two and learn how to define your goal and always draw out an action plan for the goal or venture which you may have.

Remember that your positive action to attain your goal or venture is the correct route to bringing the changes that you desire. Your reading this book from beginning to the end is part of your positive action to learn a different approach to losing weight.

The various relaxation exercises in this book will help you to relax and feel good about yourself. The various instructions about acquiring a positive mental attitude will help you to feel more positive and optimistic. This will help you in whatever you do in your attempt to lose weight, feel good, and look great day by day in every way.

Well done for reading to the end of the book.

REFERENCES

The references given below are of books which are mentioned in the text.

Descartes, Rene. 1641 *Meditations on First Philosophy*

Descartes, Rene. 1637 *Discourse on Method*

Freud, Sigmund. 1915: The Unconscious, PFL 11

Freud, Sigmund. *On Metapsychology* PFL Volume 11

Freud, Sigmund. 1916-1917: *Introductory Lectures on Psychoanalysis* PFL Vol 1

Jung, Carl Gustav. 1995: *Memories, Dreams, Reflections.*

Jung, Carl Gustav. *The Structure and Dynamics of the Psyche, Collected Works Volume 8*

Maurice-Nneke, Antony. 2023. *Stop Smoking Now!* Amazon Kendal Publications.

Maurice-Nneke, Antony. 2003. *The Psychodynamics of The Unconscious.* Intapsy Publications, London

Maurice-Nneke, Antony. 2002. *Mind Castles*. Intapsy Publications. London

Shakespeare, William. *Hamlet*